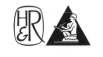

P9-AQQ-145

Alan Whiteside
and Clem Sunter

AIDS

The Challenge for South Africa

HUMAN & ROUSSEAU
TAFELBERG

First published in 2000 jointly by
Human & Rousseau (Pty) Ltd,
Design Centre, 179 Loop Street, Cape Town,
and Tafelberg Publishers Ltd,
28 Wale Street, Cape Town
© 2000 Human & Rousseau (Pty) Ltd and
Tafelberg Publishers Ltd

All rights strictly reserved. No part of this book
may be reproduced or transmitted in any form
or by any means, electronic or mechanical,
or by photocopying, recording or microfilming,
or stored in any retrieval system,
without the written permission of the publishers

Book designed by Jürgen Fomm
Charts generated by Simon Ford and
Lucy-Anne Fourie
Typeset in 10.5 on 13 pt Palatino and
printed and bound by NBD,
Drukkery Street, Goodwood, Western Cape,
South Africa

First edition, first impression 2000
ISBN 0 7981 4062 3

This book is dedicated to the thousands of people who are engaged in the fight against HIV and AIDS in South Africa. We *can* win.

It is also for Professor Brenda Gourley, the Vice Chancellor of the University of Natal, who planted the seed that led to the two of us combining our energies to make the project happen.

But most of all it is a tribute to the courage and determination of the millions of South Africans living with HIV/AIDS. Such qualities are epitomised by Lucky Mazibuko, Edwin Cameron and Mercy Makhalamele. The lives of these remarkable people offer one message: There *is* hope.

Contents

Acknowledgements

In writing this book, we received invaluable help and support from a number of people. We would like to acknowledge their input:

■ Christopher Desmond, the MSD Research Intern at the Health Economics and HIV/AIDS Research Division (HEARD) of the University of Natal, not only helped us with the research for the text but also played a key role in formulating the tables, charts, footnotes and appendices;

■ Karen Michael, also of HEARD, provided additional support in these areas;

■ Professor Alan Smith of the Department of Virology at the University of Natal, Dr Jack van Niftrik and Rose Smart, a consultant and associate of HEARD, read the manuscript and offered pertinent comments. Of course, mistakes remain our responsibility!

■ Rose Smart also provided us with initial drafts of Chapter 9 and Appendix 2. In the preparation of the latter, she was assisted by Ann Strode.

Other important contributions were made by:

■ Jan Bezuidenhout of the JD Group;

■ Dr Malcolm Steinberg and Dr Anthony Kinghorn of Abt Associates South Africa Inc. who assisted in the evolution of some of the ideas in the book;

■ Sydney Rosen, Dr Jonathan Simon, Dr Donald Thea and Dr Jeffrey R. Vincent of the Harvard Institute of International Development who developed the very perceptive tables in Chapter 8;

■ Mary Crewe of the University of Pretoria, who set us an example by writing the first book of this type on AIDS in South Africa in 1992; and

■ Dr Leon Regensberg, Dr André van Bassen and Dr Jack van Niftrik, whose treatment options provided much of the material for Appendix 1.

To Human & Rousseau, who with Tafelberg are publishing this

book, we would like to express our appreciation for printing the book in such a short period of time. In particular, we thank Kerneels Breytenbach, the General Manager: Publishing of Human & Rousseau, for giving his immediate support to the project when it was proposed; Anelma Ruschioni and Lesley Krige for co-ordinating the project; Riëtte Bothma, Magda Herbst and Linette Viljoen for general assistance; Jill Martin for editing the manuscript; and Jürgen Fomm who, together with the typesetters, printers and bookbinders, lived up to the highest standards of craftsmanship in producing this book.

We would like to pay tribute to our respective Personal Assistants, Madeline Freeman in Durban and Pat Meneghini in Johannesburg, whose habitual patience and long-suffering are appreciated in the face of countless amendments and revisions to the text.

A final word of thanks goes to our families for their forbearance and support as we tossed the manuscript to and fro and got there in the end.

Introduction

At the start of the new century, South Africa probably had the largest number of HIV-infected people of any country in the world. The only nation that comes close is India with a population of one billion people compared to our figure of 42 million. The tragedy is that this did not have to happen. South Africa was aware of the dangers posed by AIDS as early as 1985. In 1991, the national survey of women attending antenatal clinics found that only 0,8 per cent were infected. In 1994, when the new government took power, the figure was still comparatively low at 7,6 per cent. The 1999 figure which has just been published is 22,4 per cent.

This book is called *AIDS: The Challenge for South Africa*. It tracks the epidemic globally, in the region and in South Africa. We explain some of the basic concepts around the disease and look at what may happen with respect to numbers. The situation is bad, and sadly the number of people falling ill, dying and leaving families will rise over the next few years. This will impact on South Africa in a number of important ways. The book assesses the demographic, economic and social consequences of the epidemic. It disposes of a number of myths and presents the real facts.

However, as the title of the book implies, we are equally interested in spelling out the challenges facing South Africa. The message is not all bleak, for the future does not have to be like the past. HIV spread *can be prevented* and we *can deal with consequences of AIDS*. South Africa is a country which has experienced a number of miracles over the past few years. We argue that if we respond to the epidemic in the right way, not only can we reduce its impact, but perhaps we will emerge stronger as a result.

Our key message is that, along with visible leadership from government and big business, the rest is up to each and every one of us making a small contribution in our own way. The battle against HIV and AIDS will only be won by millions of initiatives at grassroots level. Some will be more effective than others, but *every little bit will count*. In the process, we have a good chance of creating a civil society – civil in the orthodox sense of building strong and sustainable institutions which are independent of the state; but civil too in the sense of instilling a genuinely caring ethic and feeling of fellowship among all the citizens who make up this remarkable country.

1 Understanding HIV and AIDS

The discovery of AIDS *and* HIV

In 1979 and 1980, doctors in the United States began to observe clusters of diseases which previously had been extremely rare. These included a type of pneumonia spread by birds (*pneumocystis carinii*) and a cancer called Karposi's sarcoma. The first public record of the phenomenon was contained in the *Morbidity and Mortality Weekly Report* (MMWR) of 5 June 1981, a widely circulated report on infectious diseases and deaths produced by the Centres for Disease Control in the USA. The MMWR recorded five cases of *pneumocystis carinii*. Later, on 3 July, the MMWR reported a clustering of cases of Karposi's sarcoma in New York. Subsequently, the number of cases of both diseases – which were mainly centred around New York and San Francisco – rose rapidly, and scientists realised that they were dealing with a new phenomenon.

Initially, most cases were seen in homosexual men. Soon, however, there was evidence of cases among haemophiliacs and recipients of blood transfusions. The disease came to be called the Acquired Immunodeficiency Syndrome, shortened to the acronym of AIDS. The name needs some explanation:

■ The 'A' stands for Acquired. This means that the virus is not spread through casual or inadvertent contact like flu or chickenpox. In order to be infected, a person has to do something (or have something done to them) which exposes them to the virus.
■ 'I' and 'D' stand for Immunodeficiency. The virus attacks a person's immune system and makes it less capable of fighting infections. Thus, the immune system becomes deficient.
■ 'S' is for Syndrome. AIDS is not just one disease but it presents itself as a number of diseases that come about as the immune system fails. Hence, it is regarded as a syndrome.

Once the new syndrome had been identified, a flurry of scientific and epidemiological activity followed. By 1983 the virus that caused AIDS had been identified by a French scientist, Luc Montagnier. Shortly thereafter, Robert Gallo, an American, also discovered the virus. It was named the Human Immunodeficiency Virus or HIV.[1] The reason it was so hard to locate is that HIV is a retrovirus, meaning that it is one of the first known viruses to transcribe DNA from an RNA template.[2] In order to exist, the virus has to enter a cell and insert itself into the cell's DNA to reproduce itself. Indeed, the first tests detected the *antibodies* to the virus rather than the virus itself. These might be compared to footprints on a sandy beach: they show that a person has been there even though that person cannot be seen. Antibodies show that a person has been (and, in the case of HIV, is) infected. Even today, most of the screening and diagnostic tests carried out are based on the discovery of the antibodies rather than the virus itself.

In 1985, a second immunodeficiency virus labelled HIV-2 was identified in humans. HIV-2 is a slower-acting virus, which appears to be found mainly in West Africa. Nevertheless, it is now slowly diffusing into other parts of the world. Insofar as HIV-1 is concerned, nine different subtypes have been discovered so far in various locations, and we are seeing an increasing spread of each variety. In southern Africa, the dominant strain is HIV-1 and, henceforth in this book, we shall refer to it as HIV.

People are said to be HIV positive when the HIV antibodies are detected in their blood. It is more difficult to define AIDS. In areas where CD4 counts and viral loads can be measured, people are regarded as having AIDS when their CD4 count falls below 200. In most settings, however, the capability to carry out such sophisticated tests does not exist. So AIDS is then defined clinically, i.e. by examining the patient and making an assessment of his or her condition. There are a number of opportunistic infections that take particular advantage of a depleted immune system, some of which are fairly unique to HIV infection. Unfortunately, TB is one disease which is increasingly seen in HIV-positive people. Complicating matters further, the new advanced drug therapies make it possible for people to move back from a state of AIDS, when they are very sick, to being HIV positive and leading normal lives again.

Does HIV cause AIDS?

There has been some questioning in South Africa of the link between HIV and AIDS in recent months. There is no debate among the vast majority of scientists, and the number who put forward these counterarguments are very few and on the fringe. The argument that HIV does not cause AIDS rests on four key elements:

1 HIV has never been isolated and identified. This is incorrect, as there are numerous photographs taken with an electron microscope of, among other things, the virus coming off the T-cell surface.
2 AIDS is a new name for old diseases and the wider spread of these diseases today is due to factors such as drug use and malnutrition and is not due to a new virus. The truth is that numerous laboratory studies and clinical research show that there is a positive correlation between the level of HIV production and viral load on the one hand and AIDS prognosis on the other. The treatments with antiretroviral therapy cause the immune system to recover, viral loads to drop and in many cases the clinical manifestations of AIDS to disappear.
3 AIDS can occur without HIV. It is true that there have been cases of immunodeficiency similar to AIDS without HIV being present. However, the number of documented cases is minute.
4 Some HIV-positive individuals do not develop AIDS. The fact is that the *average* period from infection to developing AIDS is eight to 10 years in the absence of treatment. It follows that there will be individuals who, for some reason to do with their immune system, will live for longer-than-average periods with HIV infection. Some may be fortunate to survive indefinitely without treatment. But they are exceptions – the vast majority of people will not be so fortunate and will eventually fall ill.

Obviously, dissident viewpoints cannot be ignored. For, as the great 20th-century Austrian philosopher, Karl Popper, observed, a scientific hypothesis can never be conclusively proved – only disproved. In other words, the door should always be open for conventional wisdom to be overturned. Max Planck, for example, revolutionised physics with his theory of energy coming in discrete packets. In 1900, when he put forward his theory, he was in a class of one. However, his hypothesis quickly gained credence and is now the basis of the mainstream science of quantum physics. Can the dissident school on AIDS achieve the same success?

As things stand, we believe not. Max Planck's theory took off because it explained the goings-on in the world of elementary particles better than any previous theory. In fact certain observed phenomena, such as line spectra from excited atoms, could only be explained in terms of his model. We don't think the nonviral explanation of AIDS fits the facts as well as the assumption that a virus exists. Indeed, facts like haemophiliacs dying of AIDS through tainted transfusions of blood, and this phenomenon ceasing after proper screening of blood was put in place, cannot be explained by the nonviral model.

MYTH
There is no evidence that HIV exists as a virus. Therefore it is not responsible for causing AIDS. AIDS has been around a long time and is due to factors such as poor living conditions, malnutrition, trauma and stress.
REALITY
While science can never be as certain as mathematics, the majority of the world's leading virologists believe that the HIV hypothesis is correct.

The origin of HIV

There has been a great deal of ill-informed speculation as to the source of the virus. It has been suggested that it was man-made by either the Russians or the Americans (the choice depending on the ideology of the person doing the selection!). An alternative theory is that it came from outer space. Neither of these propositions need be taken seriously.

It is now believed by scientists that HIV is a virus that crossed the species barrier into humans. It is related to a number of Simian (monkey) Immunodeficiency Viruses (SIVs) found in Africa. If the evolution of the virus is traced through a 'family tree', HIV-1 is closely related to Chimpanzee SIV and HIV-2 to Macaque SIV. Both are more distantly related to African Green Monkey SIV.

How did HIV enter the human population? An important point to note is that the spread of diseases from animals to man is not unique to HIV. Congo fever, which occurs sporadically in South Africa, is a tick-borne disease which does not kill its animal hosts, but is extremely serious when people are infected. The influenza virus, for example, evolves in birds – waterfowl to be exact.[3] The latter are what virologists call 'reservoirs' for influenza. They carry nearly all known types of influenza, with no ill effects, and spread them to the rest of the animal kingdom through their faeces. Hence, many kinds of animals can get flu – horses, ferrets, seals, pigs, among others – as well as human beings.

However, viruses can only infect and take over a cell if an appropriate 'receptor' is present. As far as we know, human beings do not have a receptor to contract avian flu directly. What is needed for human infection is for another species to act as an intermediary; it can play this role by having a receptor for avian flu and humans having a receptor for its flu. Pigs are one such species. The process can be as simple as a flu-contaminated duck dropping faeces into the dirt a pig is rolling around in, thus infecting the pig which, in turn, passes the virus on to a farmer. It can also be more complex. It is possible for a pig to be infected with one kind of flu, say human flu, only to contract another avian flu. The pig then has two types of flu simultaneously. When the pig reinfects the human, it passes on a pig-bird-human influenza. The Hong Kong Flu, for example, held seven genes from a human virus, and one gene from a duck virus, that met inside a pig to produce an entirely new hybrid.

MYTH
HIV is a unique virus inflicted on mankind as a punishment for the wicked.
REALITY
HIV is like any other virus except that it attacks the immune system itself. If only people would see that there is nothing mysterious about HIV, we could remove the stigma surrounding it and combat it more openly and effectively.

5

By comparison with other viruses, HIV is a simple virus. At some point in time, it entered the blood of humans and then spread through sexual contact from person to person. It has been suggested that the current HIV epidemic had its origin in an infection across the species barrier in the 1930s.[4] Interestingly, the transfer of the virus from an animal into a human may have happened on a number of previous occasions. However, because on those occasions each infected person did not in turn infect more than one other person, the potential epidemic petered out. There could have been a pool (or pools) of infected but isolated people in some parts of Africa for many years. What was different about the crossing of the species barriers in the 1930s (and the subsequent pattern of the epidemic) was the environment into which the virus was introduced. The upheavals of the colonial and postcolonial periods and development of a modern transport infrastructure allowed HIV to spread out into the global community very quickly.

How did the transfer from one species to another physically take place? It is not hard to imagine a hunter butchering a monkey and in the process contaminating a cut on his hand with the monkey's blood. Indeed, in February 2000, when two cases of Congo fever were reported in the North West Province, one of the virologists interviewed by the SABC warned that there was a chance that the fever could be transmitted through butchering domestic stock. Thus, it is quite possible that SIV evolved into HIV through such an event. A somewhat different explanation is given in a recent book by journalist Ed Hooper (*The River*, Penguin, London, 1999). In it, he suggests that the polio vaccination campaigns of the 1950s, during which the vaccine was cultivated on monkey kidneys, may have inadvertently spread HIV in certain populations in Central Africa.

MYTH
AIDS is the result of people having sex with monkeys.
REALITY
The disease is likely to have originated from monkeys in Africa, most probably from contact between human blood and the contaminated blood of a monkey. It is not the first, nor will it be the last, disease to cross the species barrier.

When all is said and done, the debate about the exact origin of the epidemic is academic. What matters is that the virus has reached mankind and is spreading fast.

The way the virus works

In order for infection to occur, the virus has to enter the body and attach itself to host cells (see Chart 1.1). HIV attacks a particular set of cells in the human immune system known as CD4 cells, which organise the body's overall immune response to foreign bodies and infections. These T-helper cells are the prime target of HIV. HIV also attacks immune cells called macrophages which engulf foreign invaders and ensure that the body's immune system will recognise such invaders in future. In order for a person to become infected, the virus particles (called viraemia when they are in the bloodstream) have to enter the body and attach themselves to the CD4 cells and microphages.

Chart 1.1 The virus in action[5]

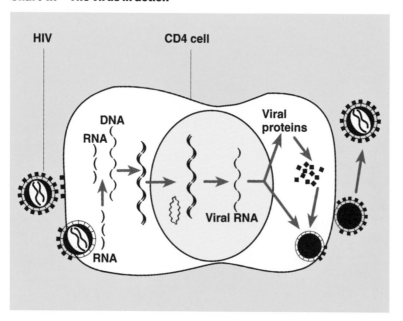

Once the virus has attached itself to the cell's surface (like the docking of a space module), it penetrates the wall. Thereafter, it is safe from the body's immune system and cannot be destroyed by the body's defence mechanisms. Inside the cell, it copies its RNA into DNA in order for the door into the cell's nucleus to be opened. There the copied DNA integrates easily into the company of the host's genes and by manipulating the proceedings of the nucleus causes the cell to churn out new HIV viral proteins. These are re-assembled into viruses which break out of the cell. In the process, the cell is destroyed and the viremia go on to infect more CD4 cells. Thus, the immune systems of infected people are gradually weakened until they fall prey to a host of diseases which they would normally fight off.

MYTH
HIV-infected individuals who show no signs of illness will not infect their partners.
REALITY
People who are HIV positive must be assumed to be infectious at all times. However, immediately after they are infected, and later, as they begin to fall ill, they are more infectious than usual because their viral load is higher.

During the early stages of infection, the antibodies to the virus (what we usually test for) may not be identifiable. This is called the 'window period'. An infected person will be very infectious during this phase. Equally, at this time a person may experience a short bout of illness. The cause is a rapid multiplication of the virus and a correspondingly rapid response from the body (see Chart 1.2). A battle commences between the virus and the immune system, described as the incubation period. During this stage, the viruses and the cells which they attack are reproducing rapidly and being destroyed as quickly by each other. Eventually, the virus is able to destroy the immune cells more quickly than they can be replaced and slowly the number of CD4 cells falls. In a healthy person, there are 1 200 CD4 cells per microlitre of blood. As the infection progresses, the number will fall to about 200 or less. At this point, new opportunistic infections begin to occur and a person is said to have AIDS. The infections will increase in frequency, severity and duration until the person dies. It is therefore the opportunistic infections that cause the syndrome referred to as AIDS.

Chart 1.2   Viral load and CD4 cell counts over time[6]

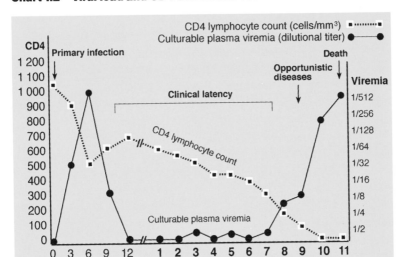

The period from HIV infection to illness and death is crucial. It is generally believed that, in the West, people will live for at least 10 years before they begin to fall ill. Without treatment, the normal period from the onset of AIDS to death was a further 12 to 24 months. Now with the development of effective antiretroviral therapies, they can expect to live a reasonable life for a longer time. Indeed, it is hoped that AIDS can be turned into a manageable, chronic disease like diabetes. In this event, people could expect to live a normal life span though they would remain infectious.

The incubation period in Africa has been estimated to be between six and eight years. The reason for shorter incubation than in the West is that, given the number of diseases in Africa, people have more challenges to their immune systems and are more vulnerable to opportunistic infection. Hence, their health deteriorates more rapidly. In addition, the period from the onset of AIDS to death is shorter – probably one year or less. The difference between Africa and the West, but also between the rich and the poor, comes down to one basic fact – people who are able to eat enough nutritious food, lead stress-free lives, and are not exposed to multiple infections will stay healthy longer.

Modes of infection

Fortunately for mankind, HIV is not a very strong virus. Every disease has a reproduction number (R_o) which is the number of other people each infected person would normally infect. In the case of HIV, R_o is around five, i.e. each HIV-positive person is likely to infect five others during his or her lifetime. The R_o for malaria, by comparison, is 100, which is the reason why it can spread so explosively. The challenge is to reduce the R_o of HIV to less than unity so that the disease goes into decline.

HIV is also hard to transmit. In order for a person to be infected, the virus has to enter the body in sufficient quantities. It must pass through an entry point in the skin and/or mucous membranes into the bloodstream. The main modes of transmission, in order of importance, are:

■ unsafe sex;
■ transmission from infected mother to child;
■ intravenous drug use with contaminated needles;
■ use of infected blood or blood products; and
■ other modes of transmission involving blood including bodily contact involving open bleeding wounds.

Sexual transmission

The vast majority of HIV infections are the result of sexual transmission. Initially in South Africa most cases were discovered among homosexual men. This was because HIV first occurred in this group in the West. Moreover, the chances of infection are higher during anal intercourse than vaginal sex. The probability of HIV infection per exposure is shown in Chart 1.3. There is a small chance that HIV can be transmitted through oral sex, especially if a person has abrasions in the mouth or gum disease such as gingivitis.

MYTH

AIDS can be got through touching and kissing, being close to an infected person and sharing facilities.

REALITY

Blood, semen, vaginal secretions or breast milk have to be involved. The chances of infection from blood spilt in the absence of contact with another person's open wound are minimal. The virus can only survive for a short period outside the human body. However, common sense dictates that contact with blood should be avoided, and people giving first aid should use protective gloves because other bloodborne diseases are more easily transmitted.

Chart 1.3   Probability of HIV-1 infection per exposure[7]

Mode of transmission	Infections per 1 000 exposures
Male-to-female, unprotected vaginal sex	1-2
Female-to-male, unprotected vaginal sex	0,33-1
Male-to-male, unprotected anal sex	5-30
Needle stick	3
Mother-to-child transmission	130-480
Exposure to contaminated blood products	900-1 000

The presence of sexually transmitted diseases (STDs), particularly ulcers or discharges, will greatly increase the odds of HIV infection. An STD means that there is more chance of the skin or membranes being broken, thus allowing the virus to enter the body. Furthermore, the very same cells that the virus is seeking to infect will be concentrated at the site of the STD because these cells are fighting the STD infection.

MYTH

Sexual intercourse with an HIV-infected person will definitely result in infection.

REALITY

HIV is a fragile virus and the chance of infection will depend on a range of factors. However, for normal healthy people, it is quite low. Women are at greater risk than men.

11

After sexual transmission, the next most important cause of HIV infection in South Africa is mother-to-child transmission (MTCT). It is known that the child can be infected with HIV prenatally, at the time of delivery or postnatally through breast-feeding. Infection at delivery is the most common mode of transmission. A number of factors influence the risk of infection, particularly the viral load of the mother at birth – the higher the load, the higher the risk. A low CD4 count is also associated with increased risk. Antiretroviral drugs may decrease the viral load and may inhibit viral reproduction in the infant, thus decreasing the risk of MTCT.

MYTH
A child born to an infected mother will be HIV positive.
REALITY
The chance of MTCT is about 30 per cent and can be greatly reduced with appropriate interventions.

There have been a number of studies into the use of antiretroviral drugs to combat MTCT in South Africa. These have been done at the Chris Hani Baragwanath Hospital in Gauteng and at King Edward Hospital in Durban. They are described in greater detail in Appendix 1, which covers treatment. Notably, however, the studies show that the chance of MTCT transmission can be greatly reduced at a relatively low cost and using fairly simple treatment regimes.

MYTH
Antiretroviral drugs are too toxic to be given to mothers and babies.
REALITY
Obviously, if you do not believe HIV exists, you can argue that no antiretroviral drugs should be given to patients because they are unnecessary as well as being toxic. However, if you do believe the virus exists, then antiretroviral drugs should be viewed in the same light as cancer drugs where their toxicity is weighed against the downside of not using them.

One issue that needs further research and clarification is that of breast-feeding. On the one hand, formula-feeding reduces the risk of MTCT; on the other hand, it increases the risk of children dying of other causes, particularly when they live in poverty. Breast-feeding has been promoted in developing countries for many years as part of child health and survival strategies. Moreover, problems with formula-feeding include the availability of the product in the short and long term; access to clean water; the means and fuel to boil the water and prepare the feed; and the knowledge of how to mix the feed. The formula approach also means that women can be 'labelled' as being HIV positive, by virtue of their using replacement feed. Recent work suggests that the key to reducing risk is consistency in either breast-feeding or formula-feeding an infant. Mixing the two is the most risky approach.

MYTH
Babies should not be saved from catching the virus because it adds to the subsequent orphan problem.
REALITY
Every life should be saved where possible. Bringing down the cost of treatment to stop MTCT is therefore a major priority.

Infection through blood and blood products

Use of contaminated blood or blood products is a very effective way of transmitting the virus, since this route introduces the virus directly into the bloodstream. This is one of the reasons why so many haemophiliacs were infected during the early years of the epidemic. They received unscreened blood products. It also accounts for early infections among recipients of blood transfusions. Fortunately, in most countries, the risks of transmission through this route are now minimal. Blood banks seek to discourage those who might be infected from donating blood, and they have the technology to test all donations. However, because of the window period when people are infected but the antibodies are not detectable, the risk of infection cannot be eliminated entirely.

13

Intravenous drug use

Drug users who share needles are at risk of infection. If the equipment is contaminated, then the virus will be introduced directly into the body. This is what has driven the epidemic in Eastern Europe and parts of Asia. Fortunately, it is not an issue in South Africa as yet.

Sport and HIV transmission[8]

The theoretical possibility of HIV transmission through open bleeding wounds in contact sports has been recognised by sports physicians. The first case of possible HIV transmission as a result of sports participation was published in 1990. This involved an Italian soccer player in whom HIV conversion was reported weeks after a traumatic incident during a soccer match. In the match, the player collided with another player who was later documented as being HIV positive. Both players sustained open bleeding wounds resulting in a possible mixing of blood. There was no indication that the first player may have been infected through any other route of HIV transmission. The authors concluded that this was the first case of HIV transmission which occurred directly as a result of participating in a sport.[9] Although this report has been criticised on epidemiological grounds, it nevertheless has clear implications for the risk of HIV transmission in sport. In particular, those people who participate in contact sports such as boxing, wrestling and rugby are potentially at risk.

There is a need to establish clear guidelines for the prevention of HIV transmission during sports participation. As early as 1989, the International Sports Medicine Federation, together with the World Health Organisation, published guidelines for the prevention of HIV transmission during contact sport.[10] Subsequently, other organisations such as the Australian Sports Medicine Federation, the American Academy of Paediatrics and the National Football League in the USA have published similar guidelines. In South Africa, the South African Football Medical Association, the South African Rugby Football Union and, most recently, the Department of Sport together with the South African Sports Medicine Association and the Department of Health have published official position statements on how to handle HIV in sport.[11]

The question that is foremost in the minds of sports administrators and participants is the risk of HIV transmission. In answer to this, there are no epidemiological data available to quantify the risk accurately. At best, a theoretical risk of transmission in a sport can be calculated by estimating the following variables:

■ the percentage prevalence of HIV among participants in a particular sport;
■ the percentage chance of an open bleeding wound being acquired by a participant in that sport;
■ the percentage chance of two players with open bleeding wounds making physical contact that could result in blood to abrasion or blood to mucous membrane exposure; and
■ the percentage chance of transmission of the virus when infected blood makes contact with an open bleeding wound (estimated to be between 0,3 and 0,5 per cent, which is similar to that calculated for a needle-stick injury in a hospital).

At present, approximate data are only available for American football in the US and professional boxing in South Africa. In American football, the HIV prevalence among players was estimated to be 0,5 per cent; the risk of an open bleeding wound 0,9 per cent and the risk of contact between players 7,7 per cent. This converts to a very low risk of transmission – one in 100 million games.

However, the odds of transmission in a boxing fight of 12 rounds in South Africa are notably higher. In a study of 952 boxers in South Africa, the HIV prevalence was determined to be nine per cent; the risk of an open bleeding wound 47 per cent and the risk of contact between boxers during a fight 100 per cent. The risk of transmission between professional South African boxers has therefore been calculated at one in 4 760 fights. The odds may be even higher because the risk of seroconversion after contact between two boxers may be greater than that of a needle-stick injury for at least two reasons: blood may be forced into the wound by the nature of the blow, and contact is usually repetitive. Of course, the risk can be greatly reduced – at the minimum by the referee not allowing a fight to continue if the seconds have not patched up a combatant's wound to his satisfaction.

Despite the lack of accurate scientific data in other contact sports, the prevention of transmission of HIV from one participant to another has to be addressed by establishing clear guidelines for the players, administrators and medical personnel involved. In rugby, for example, a player with an open wound is asked to leave the field until he has been properly stitched up. Sadly, it would appear that this rule is not as strictly applied at schools in South Africa as it should be.

Other modes of transmission

There is a possibility that HIV may be transmitted through other modes. Medical or other instruments that are contaminated can transmit the virus. Examples include dental equipment, syringes and tattoo needles. However, standard sterilisation procedures should ensure that this does not happen. Accidents through needle-stick injury or surgery are a concern for medical staff. The virus is found in all body fluids including saliva, tears and sweat, but the quantities are minute and risks of transmission are minimal. Standard precautions of using gloves and sterilising equipment will protect doctors and nurses against HIV transmission from patients (and vice versa). A source of concern is potential infection when giving first aid. Workplaces should have gloves and protective equipment available at all times. Drivers should also carry gloves in their cars in case they have to assist at the scene of an accident.

Testing

The most common HIV test is the ELISA antibody test. This is cheaper and easier to use than other screening methods. It tests for antibodies that are found in serum which has been separated from red blood cells. The serum is placed in a well containing a plastic bead coated with HIV proteins. If the test is positive, the bead will change colour. If the testing is being done for data collection and a diagnosis is not going to be given to the patient, then the ELISA test is sufficient. If, however, the testing is being done for diagnosis, and the test is positive, then it is usual for a second ELISA test to be carried out. If this is positive, then a more sophisticated test known as the Western Blot Test is usually performed. In this test, which is more expensive and complicated, the HIV proteins are laid out on a strip of film, the serum added with an enzyme, and the results read off.

A new form of test has been developed, which is noninvasive as it uses saliva. The test is cheap and easy to use, but is not accurate enough to provide diagnosis. However, it is very useful to measure HIV prevalence, especially in populations who are not prepared to give blood.

All the tests have an accuracy of over 99 per cent. They produce very few false negatives (people who are in fact HIV positive but show up as negative in the test); and even fewer false positives (people who are negative but show up as positive). Of course, people who are in the window period and have not yet developed antibodies will not test positive. This is the reason why a series of tests some months apart will be recommended for people who think they have been exposed to HIV. It is estimated that the window period can last up to six months.

MYTH
HIV tests are not accurate.
REALITY
They are extremely accurate but for the window period when people have not yet developed antibodies and will therefore test false negative.

Current prevention techniques

The first prize with any disease is to prevent it. If prevention programmes had been successful, this book would not have been written. Unfortunately, prevention has not worked in most of Africa.

The principle of successful prevention is ensuring that people are not exposed to the disease – or if they are, that they are not susceptible to infection. Vaccines provide the latter form of protection but they are not available for HIV yet. Preventing infections through blood transfusion depends on discouraging potentially infected donors from donating their blood and screening all donations. South Africa has as safe a supply of blood and blood products as science can make it. Occupational exposure can be reduced through adopting universally accepted precautions regarding safety and sterility. In the event that a health-care worker is exposed, immediate treatment with antiretroviral therapy can greatly reduce the risk of an infection becoming established. Fortunately, drug use by injection is not a big issue in South Africa at present; but again simple procedures such as the use of sterilised needles and needle exchange programmes have been shown to be very successful.

Preventing sexual transmission

As sex is the main mode of transmission, it is here that winning prevention strategies are needed. One of the first responses to the epidemic was to call for isolation of HIV-infected people. This was seen in most quarters around the globe as unimplementable and discriminatory. The one exception is Cuba which in the 1980s tested the entire population and isolated those found to be HIV positive in 'sanatoria'. This has probably contributed to the low level of HIV infection seen to date in that country. At the end of 1997, it was estimated that there were only 1 400 infected Cubans.[12] However, for this approach to work, a high degree of governmental control is necessary, and everyone entering the country has to be tested. In addition, there needs to be a regular repeat testing programme for the local population. This was never an option for any African country and certainly not for South Africa. Apart from the expense and difficulty in implementing such a programme, there are concerns that it is a gross violation of human rights.

In order to prevent sexual transmission there is a limited, but potentially effective, range of interventions. The first set of interventions are 'biomedical'. These aim to ensure that if a person has sex with someone who is infected, then the risk is reduced. Good sexual health is paramount. This means that STDs should be treated immediately, and the availability of STD treatment in the developed world has probably played a major role in controlling HIV. Sexual practices which increase risk should be discouraged: an example in South Africa is 'dry sex', where a woman uses a drying agent in the vagina before intercourse in the belief that it gives more pleasure. The reality is that it increases the risk of tears and abrasions, and therefore facilitates the entry of the virus.

The most effective intervention is the use of condoms. Condoms provide a barrier to the virus and, if properly used, are effective. There are both male and female condoms available. Male condoms can be purchased at many retail outlets and cost about R1,50 each. However, at some sites, they are provided free (or at much reduced cost) by the state, by employers or by NGOs engaged in prevention campaigns. Female condoms are more expensive, costing R3 each, and are more difficult to use. However, because many men refuse to wear condoms, female condoms represent an important alternative as a safety measure for women.

MYTH
Condoms don't work because the virus can pass though the latex, and anyway they fail.
REALITY
The virus cannot pass through the latex. If condoms are used properly, consistently, and are SABS (South African Bureau of Standards) approved, they provide close to 100 per cent protection.

The second set of interventions are those that seek to prevent people from being exposed to HIV by altering their sexual behaviour. These are the knowledge, attitude and behaviour (KAB) interventions. First, people need to have *knowledge,* then change their *attitudes* and finally alter their *behaviour.* People are encouraged to stick to one partner, delay the first experience of sexual intercourse, and use condoms if they have more than one partner. This is the classic ABC message: A – abstain; B – be faithful; C – condom if necessary.

The problem is that, even if people have the knowledge, they may not have the incentive or the power to change their behaviour. This is illustrated in Chart 1.4, which shows how the epidemic is being driven (and where current interventions are).

The chart indicates that, although the most proximate causes of being infected are biological, a person's sexual behaviour is next in line as it determines the number and type of sexual encounters he or she will have. Sexual behaviour is in turn determined by econom-

Chart 1.4   HIV epidemic – determinants

DETERMINANTS

Macro factors	Socio-economic environment	Sexual behaviour	Biomedical	HIV INFECTION
Wealth	Migration	Rate of partner change	Virus subtypes	AIDS
Income distribution	Mobility	Concurrent partners	Stage of infection	
Culture	Urbanisation	Sexual mixing patterns	Presence of other STDs	
Religion	Access to health care	Sexual practices	Gender	
Governance	Levels of violence		Circumcision	
	Women's rights and status			

INTERVENTIONS

		Behaviour change	STD treatment	
		- fewer partners - delay intercourse - condom use	Condom availability	

ic, social and cultural factors. For example, a truck driver on the Durban-Johannesburg-Durban run might have sex with a commercial sex worker because he is bored; he feels his job is dangerous and he deserves some compensation; he is frequently away from his wife and family; he experiences peer pressure from his fellow drivers to engage in this activity; and he has the necessary money. The commercial sex worker, on the other hand, is driven by poverty and the need to feed her family.

Chart 1.4 suggests that, for successful control of the epidemic, interventions are required that address the socio-economic environment and make it possible for people to change their behaviour. Current interventions in South Africa constitute a *necessary condition* for control but are not a *sufficient condition*. This was recognised by the Department of Health's Beyond Awareness Campaign. If prevention is to move beyond knowledge to action, we must look at the socio-economic causes of the epidemic and intervene there too. In the end, there is no magic bullet and the only way to prevent the epidemic spreading is to institute a variety of measures which tackle the different links in the causal chain that leads to transmission of the virus.

Treatment[13]

HIV is the most intensively studied disease ever. Much research has gone into the search for a cure and a vaccine. Neither has been developed yet. However, there have been major advances in medical treatment. Three of the programmes currently available in South Africa are more fully described in Appendix 1 at the back of the book.

The developments in treatment have resulted in a decline in the mortality rates from HIV in the developed world. There are three stages in the treatment of HIV-positive people. The first is when they are infected, but CD4 cell counts are high. At this point, the emphasis is on 'positive living' – staying healthy, eating the correct food and so on. The second stage is when the CD4 cell count begins to drop. At this stage, prophylactic treatment to prevent TB and other common diseases is normally begun. The third stage is the use of antiretroviral drugs to fight HIV directly. This can start when the CD4 cell count drops below 350.

Since the first antiretroviral drugs were developed, many new generations of drugs are becoming available. At the moment antiretroviral drugs may be used in single therapies (just one drug), double therapies (a combination of two drugs) or triple therapies (three drugs). The way the drugs act is shown in Chart 1.5. Single-drug therapy is by and large no longer used because it can cause fairly swift mutation of the virus into drug-resistant strains. However, single drugs are administered as a prophylaxis to stop mother-to-child transmission. Dual therapy is cheaper than triple therapy, but the antiviral effect is less immediate as the viral load falls slowly and the viral control may be of a limited duration. Highly Active Antiretroviral Therapy (HAART) is any antiretroviral regimen capable of suppressing HIV for many months and perhaps years in a significant number of individuals. Such is the case with triple therapy. It usually involves the use of two reverse transcriptase inhibitors and one protease inhibitor. Although not a cure, such treatments are highly effective in rapidly reducing the viral load to undetectable levels, thereby prolonging survival.

MYTH

AIDS is untreatable.

REALITY

Therapies are available which reduce viral load (and therefore infectiousness). They definitely improve the quality of life of people living with AIDS, but the challenge is to make them affordable to everyone.

The issue of timing for introducing a HAART regimen is of some importance. Early treatment prevents damage to the body caused by high and prolonged viral loads – but it does use up the big guns sooner (which can decrease subsequent options if resistance builds up). That is why for long-term patients some doctors prefer to step up the treatment gradually, starting with dual-drug therapy. Cost is also a factor with dual-drug therapy priced at between R15 000 and R25 000 a year, compared to a triple-drug regime lying between R35 000 and R50 000 a year.[14] The latter range is still valid despite the devaluation of the rand and is well below the figure of R70 000 (i.e. $10 000 times seven) bandied around in the press. At present, most medical aid schemes cap their AIDS expenditure at R15 000 to R25 000 per patient per annum. This usually permits single- and double-drug therapy, but special dispensation has to be sought for triple-drug therapy. Of course, for the majority of AIDS sufferers with no medical aid, all these treatments are out of reach.

Getting patients to adhere to a complicated pill-taking programme is also a real problem. Some triple-drug therapies involve taking 18 pills a day in a particular sequence. Yet adherence to prescribed anti-HIV drug regimens is crucial for long-term success. Missing a single dose of medication may allow drug concentration in blood and tissues to drop below that needed for full HIV suppression. This decrease allows HIV replication to occur in the optimum environment for selection of drug-resistant mutant strains. Combination pills are at present being developed to make adherence easier.

Chart 1.5   Where the drugs act

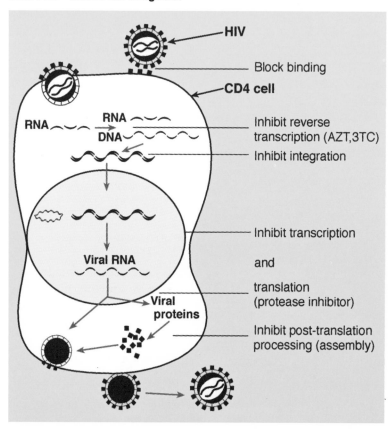

Vaccine

Intensive research is being carried out to develop a vaccine with varying degrees of success. More than 15 years have passed since the first efforts, but as yet a vaccine remains elusive. Unfortunately the amount of money spent on researching AIDS vaccines is small ($300-600 million a year) and is focused on strains found mainly in the US and Western Europe. The World Bank and the European Union, among others, have been involved in the search for new mechanisms and incentives to increase research and development for vaccines for developing countries. The International AIDS Vaccine Initiative (IAVI), based in New York, plays an increasingly important role in mustering resources and facilitating development.

The South African AIDS Vaccine Initiative (SAAVI) was launched in 1999, with support from the highest levels in the South African government. The R20 million programme, headed by Dr Walter Prozesky, is working with IAVI and other partners to encourage South African vaccine development efforts. The (optimistic) aim is to develop an effective, affordable preventive vaccine for universal use in South Africa and the Southern African Development Community (SADC) by 2005. Eskom has recently announced that it is contributing R30 million towards this programme. The first trials will be in the Hlabisa district of KwaZulu-Natal.

MYTH
Recent medical advances mean that AIDS can be cured.
REALITY
Although the medical advances have been spectacular, there is still no cure or vaccine for AIDS. What we know is that taking various combinations of drugs can reduce the virus to undetectable levels. However, this does not work for all patients. There are side effects; compliance is not easy; the virus develops resistance to some drugs in some patients; and it is probable that once people stop taking the drugs, the virus particles will rebound. The drugs are also very expensive at present, although there is a good chance that the prices will come down.

HIV and other diseases[15]

As the immune system is depressed by HIV, other diseases will affect HIV-positive people. Most of these are not a threat to uninfected people. For example, people with HIV are very much more likely to develop active TB. In the absence of HIV, the chance of developing TB is low and is estimated at 10 per cent in a lifetime. In the event that the person is co-infected with HIV, the chance rises to 5-10 per cent per year. It is estimated that 40-50 per cent of people in South Africa with TB are co-infected with HIV, and one third of people with HIV are expected to contract TB. This has to be seen against a background of very high levels of new cases of TB in

South Africa. The annual incidence per 100 000 people between 1996 and 1998 was 254. In Europe it is 19, China 113 and India 187.

TB can be treated. For instance, the DOTS regime (Directly Observed Treatment, Short course) has seen cure rates rise from 50 to 57 per cent from 1995 to 1997. But this is for all patients. Prophylactic treatment for HIV-positive people is far more costly and problematic. Not for nothing are HIV and TB variously referred to as 'the terrible twins' and 'Bonnie and Clyde'. The same applies to HIV and malaria.

2 The basic epidemiology and data sources

Epidemiology has been defined as 'the study of the distribution and the determinants of states of health in populations, with the objective of prevention and controlling ill health'.[1] In other words, while the last chapter dealt with details of the virus itself, this chapter is concerned with the broader impact of HIV and AIDS on the population at large.

Epidemic curves

Epidemics usually follow an 'S' curve as shown in Chart 2.1. They start slowly and gradually. At a certain stage, a critical mass of infected people is reached and the growth of new infections thereafter accelerates. The epidemic then spreads through the population until many of those who are susceptible to infection have been infected. Some are lucky because even though they are susceptible, they never come into contact with an infectious person. This was the case with the bubonic plague which wiped out between a third and a half of Europe's population in the 14th century. The disease was spread by fleas on rats. Many of the people who survived the plague lived in relatively isolated communities. With modern means of transport, instances of isolated communities are rarer. Hence, epidemics can go global much more quickly and affect more people, particularly in light of the much greater number alive in the world today.

In the final phase of an epidemic – where the 'S' flattens off at the top – people are either getting better or deaths outnumber new cases so that the total number alive and infected passes its peak and begins to decline. With most diseases the curve will decline rapidly. HIV and AIDS are different.

What sets HIV and AIDS apart from other epidemics is that there are two curves, as shown in the chart. The HIV one precedes the AIDS one by about six to eight years, reflecting the incubation period between first being infected and the onset of illness. This is

Chart 2.1   The two epidemic curves

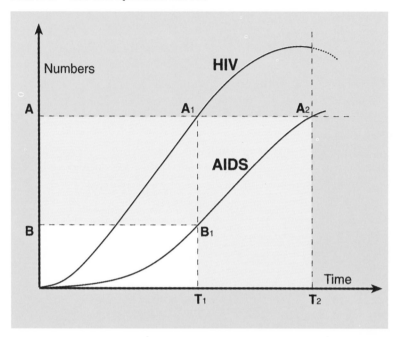

why HIV is such a lethal epidemic compared to, say, cholera. In the latter case, victims of the disease die quickly, which puts the general population and public health professionals on their guard. They take precautions to halt the spread of the disease. In the case of HIV, however, the epidemic is silently and stealthily creeping through the population and it is only later – when the HIV pool has risen to a considerable level – that the true impact of the epidemic is felt in terms of AIDS deaths. By then, the epidemic is in full swing and the only way people leave the pool of infections is by dying, since there is no cure yet. Chart 2.1 illustrates this point clearly. The vertical axis represents numbers and the horizontal axis time. At T_1, when the level of HIV is at A_1, the number of AIDS cases will be very much lower at B_1. The AIDS cases will only reach A_2 (i.e. the same level as A_1) at T_2. A considerable amount of time will have elapsed and HIV will have risen even higher, though it may be levelling off.

27

The second conclusion to be drawn from the chart is that, while prevention efforts may aim to lower the number of new infections, the reality is that – without affordable and effective treatment – AIDS will still be increasing long after the HIV tide has been turned.

MYTH

If there was a genuine HIV epidemic in South Africa, we should now be seeing people dying in droves in the streets.

REALITY

Without treatment, people will only start dying in large numbers some years from now (although parts of South Africa are seeing a rise in mortality). Moreover, because people will be dying of the many opportunistic infections brought on by AIDS, the true impact of the epidemic will remain camouflaged and largely invisible. Anyway, we should never expect people to die on the street.

Incidence and prevalence

Incidence and prevalence are two important concepts to grasp when looking at HIV/AIDS data (and indeed any data on disease). *Incidence* is the number of new infections over a given period of time. The *incidence rate* is the number per specified unit of population (this can be per 1 000, per 10 000 or per million for rare diseases). *Prevalence* is the absolute number of people infected. The *prevalence rate* is the percentage of the population which exhibits the disease at a particular time (or averaged over a period of time). A numerical example and an illustration are given in Charts 2.2 and 2.3 respectively.

Chart 2.2   Incidence and prevalence

Year	Population	Incidence (actual)	Incidence rate per 1 000	Prevalence	Prevalence rate (per cent)
1	9 750	0	0	0	0
2	10 000	50	5	50	0,5
3	10 500	50	4,7	100	1,0
4	11 000	150	13,6	250	2,3
5	12 000	750	62,5	1 000	8,3

28

The key statistics for tracking the course of the HIV epidemic are the incidence rate and the prevalence rate. With HIV, prevalence rates are given as a percentage of a specific segment of the population, e.g. children below the age of five, adults aged between 15 and 65, antenatal clinic attenders, blood donors, men with STDs, or the 'at risk' population, taken to mean 15- to 49-year-olds who are sexually active. HIV is unique in that it is the only disease where prevalence is given as a percentage rather than a rate. It is crucial to establish what the denominator is when the percentage is quoted. HIV and AIDS incidence is normally given as the rate per 1 000.

Chart 2.3   HIV and AIDS incidence and prevalence

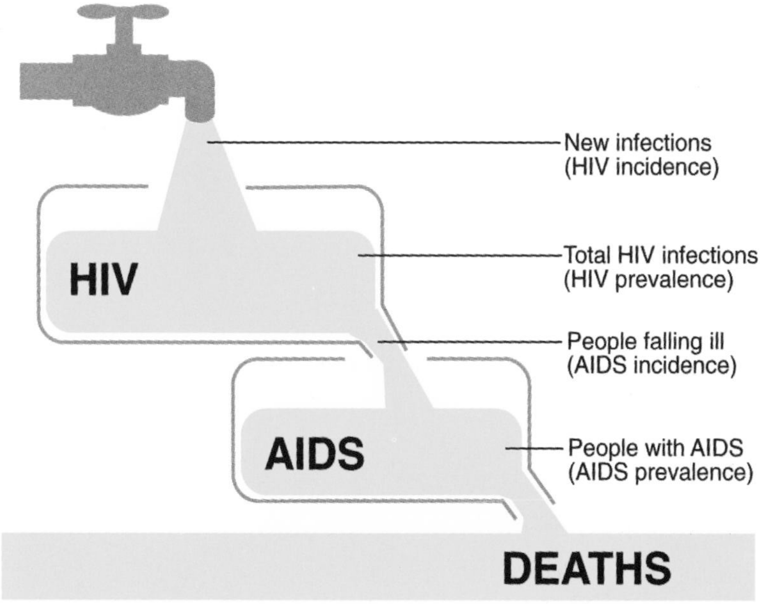

New infections
(HIV incidence)

Total HIV infections
(HIV prevalence)

People falling ill
(AIDS incidence)

People with AIDS
(AIDS prevalence)

HIV

AIDS

DEATHS

Note: The only point at which measurements are regularly made is HIV prevalence

Annual incidence is normally calculated by subtracting the previous year's from the current year's prevalence. Unfortunately, because we don't know when people were actually infected – we only know the date on which we *discover* they are infected – the data which would be most helpful in measuring the impact of prevention efforts

29

are simply not available. Moreover, high incidence may occur even when prevalence has levelled off, because those dying are being replaced by newly infected people.

Data sources

Epidemiological data are usually drawn from official sources. The two most common types of data are AIDS case data and HIV data.

AIDS case data

In the early years of the epidemic, AIDS case data were what hit the headlines. Unfortunately, the press often fails to distinguish between HIV and AIDS. As recently as 23 March 2000, *The Star's* headline was 'Hope for babies from moms with AIDS' while the first paragraph of the article (which concerned treatment with nevirapine) read: 'Pregnant women who are HIV positive could soon have access to a drug which will halve the risk of their babies contracting the virus.' Of course, the article uses HIV correctly and the headline is misleading.

Where AIDS case data are reported, the number of cases is usually analysed by age, gender and type of transmission. In African countries, most AIDS cases are not officially recorded. There are a number of reasons for this:

■ Reporting may be very slow. It takes time for data to flow into a central point and be collated.

■ Data may be inaccurate because of the unwillingness of medical staff to report cases. This may be due to the stigma associated with AIDS or medical aid societies and insurance companies paying out more for other diseases.

■ AIDS may not be the condition diagnosed; instead the patient may be recorded as having TB or meningitis.

■ Doctors may feel that it is pointless to report cases as there are always problems with collecting and collating the data.

In many developing countries, one of the principal stumbling blocks to cases being reported is that most people are not seen by the formal medical services.

The process a person with AIDS would have to go through to be officially recorded as having the disease is illustrated in Chart 2.4. Alongside are all the things that can go wrong.

Chart 2.4   The problems of AIDS case reporting

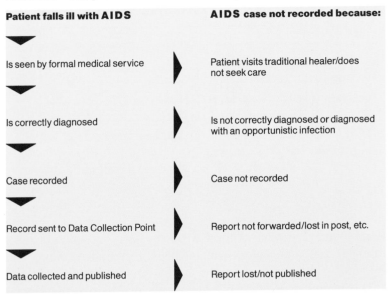

Patient falls ill with AIDS	AIDS case not recorded because:
Is seen by formal medical service	Patient visits traditional healer/does not seek care
Is correctly diagnosed	Is not correctly diagnosed or diagnosed with an opportunistic infection
Case recorded	Case not recorded
Record sent to Data Collection Point	Report not forwarded/lost in post, etc.
Data collected and published	Report lost/not published

As indicated in the discussion on the epidemic curves, the AIDS cases recorded at any given time (even if this is done accurately) reflect the HIV infections of six or more years earlier. AIDS cases are no longer recorded in South Africa, although there have been moves to reintroduce the practice.

More than a year ago a new death certificate was introduced. It tried to provide a balance between privacy and the need for epidemiological information. The certificate comprises two parts, which are later separated. The first is the public document and provides the information for legal matters, i.e. natural or unnatural deaths, and does not indicate which are AIDS deaths. The second part is an epidemiological form, which is aimed at providing statistics to monitor the path of the epidemic. The two parts are not linked. Despite its introduction, no information appears to be forthcoming. Reasons for this include information problems, as health practition-

31

ers appear to be largely unaware of the change. The collection process also appears not to be working, with the result that no data are being produced.

Chart 2.5   Distribution of AIDS cases by age and gender 1995[2]

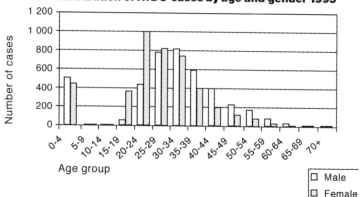

What then is the value of these AIDS case data? A graph of AIDS cases by age and gender can be helpful in understanding the epidemic. This is shown in Chart 2.5 for South Africa.

The figures show that the first group of cases occurs among infants and children. These are the cases that result from mother-to-child transmission. The next clustering of cases is in adults aged between 25 and 45, with women being infected and falling ill earlier than men. What these graphs (and they are virtually identical in shape for all African countries) also show is a small number of cases in older children and young teenagers. This is indicative, on the one hand, of the small number of children who survive beyond five years with HIV; but, on the other hand, it demonstrates the existence of child abuse, something that has not been admitted in African society before now.

AIDS case data can also be misinterpreted. The classic example comes from Swaziland where there has been a huge public debate over the number of infected Swazi. The problem stems from a statement in the 1998 Surveillance Report which says: 'When using the WHO guideline that for each case of AIDS reported there could be 100 individuals living with HIV and taking into account that by

March 1998 there were 2 931 cases reported to the Ministry of Health and Social Welfare (cumulatively from 1987), it is estimated there could now be as many as 293 100 people living with HIV in the country, which is approximately 30 per cent of the total population.'[3]

The truth is that there is no such WHO guideline and the figure of HIV infections in Swaziland was greatly overstated (as the discussion on HIV data will shortly demonstrate).

HIV data

HIV data in South Africa are drawn from surveys of specific groups. In the early years of the epidemic they included blood donors, STD clinic attenders, people with TB and women attending antenatal clinics. A number of surveys were done of commercial sex workers and truck drivers as well. Today, the consistent data come from the antenatal clinic surveys.

In trying to establish what was happening in the epidemic, the scientists needed a sample which was broadly representative of the general population. In addition, they required one that they could draw on at regular intervals, usually every year or two. Antenatal clinic attenders provide a good sample because they are sexually active and adult. Another advantage is that blood is routinely taken from women attending these clinics for a number of standard tests and, until recently, the only way to test for HIV was through blood.

The way antenatal HIV surveys are done is that every year a sample of women attending the state antenatal clinics have a portion of their blood sent for testing. This is done on an anonymous, unlinked basis. In other words, any given woman cannot be identified as having given a certain sample. This means that informed consent is not needed. In South Africa the annual survey is carried out in October/November of each year, and each sample is labelled with the location and age of that woman. A small amount of other information, such as marital status or income, can be collected without compromising confidentiality. There are biases: younger women will be overrepresented as they are more sexually active and likely to fall pregnant; and HIV-positive women will be underrepresented as HIV infection reduces fertility.

MYTH

We don't have any idea how big (or small) the HIV epidemic is in Africa.

REALITY

Recent population-based studies have shown that antenatal clinic data do provide a good estimate of HIV prevalence in adults aged 15 to 49. When the epidemic is modelled, the data are manipulated to produce estimates of prevalence for all adults and for the population at large.

An obvious drawback to the present method of sampling is that it applies solely to women attending the state antenatal clinics. It does not cover the general population or even better-off women who attend private gynaecologists. Nonetheless, once the raw data from the state antenatal clinics are available, it is possible to estimate the percentage of all women, men and adults who are infected, as well as the percentage of children who will be born HIV positive. This is done using a model which adjusts for:

■ The degree to which antenatal clinic attendance figures are un-representative due to the adverse impact of HIV on fertility of women.

■ The fact that there are young and old members of both sexes who are not (or not as) sexually active.

■ The lower prevalence in men.

■ The number of children expected to be infected through mother-to-child transmission.

The raw data can then be turned into more representative numbers, using various computer models. Some of these are in the public domain, which means that anyone can download them from the Internet and use them.[4] But there remains a danger of statisticians producing figures with an appearance of great accuracy. Precision in the field of HIV and AIDS is *spurious!* We do not know exactly how many people are infected and will fall ill and die – or when. We make estimates; and the better the data we start with, the more comfortable we will be with the estimates. But they remain just that – *estimates.*

To return to the Swaziland data again, the 1998 survey found that 31,6 per cent of women attending the clinics at the time of the survey were infected.[5] The report then estimated that HIV prevalence among the Swazi population aged between 15 and 49 was 23 per cent. Given Swaziland's demographic structure, the percentage of the total population infected might be about 14 per cent. Hence, based on a total population of about 978 200 in 1997, it would seem that the total number of infected Swazis would have been about 130 000 or less than half the figure quoted in the 1998 Surveillance Report.

Antenatal clinic data are appropriate when the epidemic is largely heterosexually driven, as is the case in Africa and most of Asia. It may not be appropriate where the majority of cases are men who have sex with men, or injecting drug users. In this situation, other data will need to be collected.[6]

MYTH

AIDS experts exaggerate the scale of the epidemic to ensure that they remain employed.

REALITY

Because most samples are limited, there is an irreducible level of uncertainty about all HIV and AIDS figures. One of the priorities, therefore, of those working in the field is to collect better data. From what we know, however, we do have cause for alarm.

Clearly, in South Africa, a better method of assessing the HIV status of the general population would be to sample it directly. However, people are reluctant to give blood for survey purposes and such surveys would also be expensive. The recent development of tests that will detect HIV antibodies in saliva may well change this. It has to be said, though, that the latter tests are accurate for *surveying* but not for *diagnosis*. Before an HIV or AIDS diagnosis is given, confirmatory testing is required.

3 The global epidemic[1]

In 1998, when UNAIDS issued a map showing global infections, the caption was: 'No place on earth untouched'. This is certainly the case; but what is also evident is that some parts of the world are worse affected than others. Chart 3.1 summarises the global position at the end of 1999. In terms of the definitions we gave in the last chapter, the first row of the chart represents global incidence and the second row combined HIV and AIDS prevalence.

Chart 3.1   Global summary of the HIV/AIDS epidemic, December 1999

People newly infected with HIV in 1999	Total	5,6 million
	Adults	5 million
	Women	*2,3 million*
	Children < 15 years	570 000 million
Number of people living with HIV/AIDS	Total	33,6 million
	Adults	32,4 million
	Women	*14,8 million*
	Children < 15 years	1,2 million
AIDS deaths in 1999	Total	2,6 million
	Adults	2,1 million
	Women	*1,1 million*
	Children < 15 years	470 000
Total number of AIDS deaths since the beginning of the epidemic	Total	16,3 million
	Adults	12,7 million
	Women	*6,2 million*
	Children < 15 years	3,6 million

In 1999, there were 2,6 million deaths from HIV/AIDS. This was a higher global total than in any year since the beginning of the epidemic, despite antiretroviral therapy which staved off AIDS and

AIDS deaths in the richer countries. Even in a scenario where prevention programmes managed to cut the number of new infections to zero, deaths among those already infected would continue mounting for some years. However, with the HIV-positive population still expanding – there were 5,6 million new infections in 1999 compared to 2,6 million deaths – the annual number of AIDS deaths can be expected to increase substantially for many more years.

Around half of all people who acquire HIV become infected before they turn 25 and typically die before their 35th birthday. This age factor makes AIDS uniquely threatening to the bringing-up of children. Most people will have had children before they become infected, and about 70 per cent of children born to infected mothers will not, themselves, be infected. These children have a close to 100 per cent chance of being orphaned. By the end of 1999, the epidemic had left behind a cumulative total of 11,2 million AIDS orphans (defined as those having lost their mother before reaching the age of 15). Many of these maternal orphans have also lost their father.

Also of significance in the global data is that the number of women infected is increasing. Within the next year or so, there will be more women infected than men. This is already the case in most of Africa.

MYTH

AIDS is a disease which is mainly restricted to the homosexual community.

REALITY

In the near future, it is likely that more women in the world will be HIV positive than men. This is because the chances of transmission from an HIV-positive man to an HIV-free women are considerably higher than vice versa. In addition, a range of social, cultural and gender factors increase the likelihood that women will be infected.

Global diversity

The epidemic is not the same all over the world. The overwhelming majority of people with HIV – some 95 per cent of the global total – live in the developing world. That proportion is set to grow even

37

further as infection rates continue to rise in countries where poverty, poor health systems, lack of education, inequality and limited resources for prevention and care fuel the spread of the virus. The diversity between different continents is illustrated in Chart 3.2. The main message, though, is that currently sub-Saharan Africa dwarfs the rest.

Chart 3.2   Regional HIV/AIDS statistics and features, December 1999

Region	Epidemic started	Adults & children living with HIV/AIDS (prevalence)	Adults & children newly infected with HIV in 1999 (incidence)	Adult prevalence rate (per cent)	Proportion of HIV-positive adults who are women (per cent)	Main mode(s) of transmission for adults living with HIV/AIDS
Sub-Saharan Africa	late '70s - early '80s	23,3 million	3,8 million	8,0	55	Hetero
North Africa & Middle East	late '80s	220 000	19 000	0,13	20	IDU, Hetero
South & South-East Asia	late '80s	6 million	1,3 million	0,69	30	Hetero
East Asia & Pacific	late '80s	530 000	120 000	0,07	15	IDU, Hetero, MSM
Latin America	late '70s - early '80s	1,3 million	150 000	0,57	20	MSM, IDU, Hetero
Caribbean	late '70s - early '80s	360 000	57 000	1,96	35	Hetero, MSM
Eastern Europe & Central Asia	early '90s	360 000	95 000	0,14	20	IDU, MSM
Western Europe	late '70s - early '80s	520 000	30 000	0,25	20	MSM, IDU
North America	late '70s - early '80s	920 000	44 000	0,56	20	MSM, IDU, Hetero
Australia & New Zealand	late '70s - early '80s	12 000	500	0,1	10	MSM, IDU
TOTAL		33,6 million	5,6 million	1,1	46	

Note that:

■ The adult prevalence rate in the fourth column is the proportion of adults (15 to 49 years of age) living with HIV/AIDS in 1999, using 1998 population numbers as the denominator.

■ In the last column, MSM stands for sexual transmission among men who have sex with men; IDU stands for transmission through drug use by injection; Hetero stands for heterosexual transmission.

38

MYTH

1. South Africa will follow the industrialised countries' pattern.
2. Asia will experience an African-scale epidemic.

REALITY

South Africa already has an epidemic many times larger than that experienced by the worst-hit industrialised country. Early evidence suggests that parts of Asia may experience a similar epidemic to Africa, but there will be considerable differences across the continent. Different countries have different epidemic patterns. This implies that different preventive programmes, suitably tailored for local conditions and the predominant mode of transmission in a particular country, should be implemented.

Industrialised countries

In industrialised countries, the epidemic is largely under control. The numbers of new cases of AIDS, and AIDS deaths, have fallen significantly because of the availability of antiretroviral therapy for most of those diagnosed. However, the rate at which AIDS deaths have been falling over the last three years is beginning to taper off, suggesting that current therapies have limited effectiveness. In the United States, for example, AIDS deaths decreased by 42 per cent between 1996 and 1997, but by only half that proportion between 1997 and 1998. In Western Europe, deaths fell by 20 per cent in 1999, a significantly smaller reduction than in the previous year.

There is some evidence to suggest that HIV infections among those at particular risk are increasing. These include drug users and other marginalised groups. A new development reported by UNAIDS is 'that the advent of life-prolonging therapies may have led to complacency about the dangers of HIV, and that that complacency may be leading to rises in risky behaviour. A study in the US city of San Francisco, for example, showed that in 1993-1994 just over one-third of gay men reported having had unprotected anal intercourse, while the proportion of men reporting anal sex without a condom rose to one-half three years later, when effective death-postponing therapy had become available. Many of these men did not know their partners' HIV status'.[2]

What makes this all the more worrying, in a population with

39

historically high-risk behaviour, is that the absolute number of HIV-positive people is probably growing because they are surviving longer with antiretroviral drugs. Although antiretroviral therapy should reduce a person's infectiousness – the likelihood that he or she will pass on the virus to a sex partner – this effect should not be taken to mean that there is no risk of infection. For now, it must be assumed on the contrary that a higher level of HIV in the pool of potential sex partners means a higher risk of transmission whenever there is unprotected sex with a partner of unknown HIV status.

UNAIDS/WHO estimate that some 1,5 million people were living with HIV in the West (defined as North America, Western Europe, Australia and New Zealand) at the end of 1999.

Eastern Europe

The world's steepest HIV curve in 1999 was recorded in the newly independent states of the former Soviet Union, where the proportion of the population living with HIV doubled between end-1997 and end-1999. Data indicate that the majority of new infections were among injecting drug users and most occurred in the Ukraine and the Russian Federation. The rapid growth is illustrated in Chart 3.3.

Chart 3.3   Detected HIV among total pupulation and intravenous drug users (IVDUs) in Ukraine 1992-1996[3]

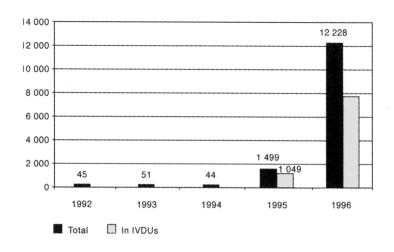

The Middle East

In the Middle East, the level of reported infection is low. It seems that the epidemic is being driven by drug use by injection. This form of transmission accounts for two-thirds of reported cases in Bahrain in 1998 and half in the Islamic Republic of Iran. In Tunisia, injecting drug use is responsible for more than one-third of AIDS cases. In Egypt, one AIDS case in 10 is among drug injectors. In Pakistan, 5,4 per cent of 703 drug injectors tested HIV positive in 1995.

The scale of drug use will determine the future course of the epidemic. Recent studies by the United Nations International Drug Control Programme in a few countries of the Middle East – Egypt, Iran and Lebanon – indicate that the magnitude of the drug-abuse problem should not be underestimated.

The region also has a problem of sexually transmitted diseases, particularly among young adults and in urban areas. However, the reporting of cases is low.

Latin America

The main feature of Latin America over the past few years has been the introduction of antiretroviral treatment for people infected with HIV. Brazil spent some US$ 300 million in 1999, providing drugs for around 75 000 people. The argument made by health officials is that savings on episodes of hospitalisation and medical care for patients justify the cost of the drugs. This, along with weak surveillance systems, make it difficult to gain a clear picture of the epidemic's trend. However, rates of infection are generally low outside the groups with the highest risk behaviour. In 1999 in Argentina, for example, just under three pregnant women in 1 000 tested positive for HIV; while even among people with STDs – usually considered a high-risk group for HIV infection – rates were below seven per 1 000. In Uruguay, similarly low rates were recorded from a sample of over 8 000 workers tested in 1997, with less than three per 1 000 testing positive for HIV.

Central America and the Caribbean

In this region infections are on the rise. In Guatemala in 1999, some two to four per cent of pregnant women tested at antenatal clinics in major urban areas were found to have HIV. Indeed, the Caribbean basin has some of the worst HIV epidemics outside of sub-Saharan Africa. In Guyana, HIV prevalence was recorded at 3,2 per cent in blood donors – who are generally thought to represent a population at low risk of infection – while screening of urban sex workers in 1997 showed 46 per cent were infected. The last time Haiti performed HIV surveillance among pregnant women, in 1996, close to six per cent tested positive for the virus. Infection rates approaching eight per cent had already been registered in some antenatal clinics as early as 1993.

Asia

The picture in Asia is mixed. In some countries the epidemic appears to be under control. These include the Philippines, Malaysia and Sri Lanka. In Bangladesh, Indonesia, Vietnam, Nepal and Pakistan the prevalence rates are low but there are indications that they could rise as HIV spreads out from drug users and commercial sex workers.

Elsewhere there appear to be some serious and growing epidemics. In Myanmar, HIV infections are high and rising, but no recent data are available. Asia's highest levels of infection continue to be recorded in Cambodia, where surveillance suggests that HIV is well established in the general population in all provinces. HIV prevalence among pregnant women in 1998 exceeded two per cent in 12 out of the country's 19 provinces. Nationally, on average, some 3,7 per cent of married women of reproductive age were HIV positive in 1998. At the moment, prevalence in men may be somewhat higher – 4,5 per cent of male blood donors were infected with HIV compared with 2,5 per cent of female donors.

The huge populations of India and China mean that they dominate assessments of HIV in Asia. India has recently made a major effort to improve its understanding of the HIV epidemic. As one would expect in a country as vast and diverse as India, the situation is extremely variable. Overall there are thought to be about four million Indians infected. In some states, principally in the south and west of the country, HIV has a significant grip on the urban population, with over one pregnant woman in 50 testing positive for HIV. In the north-east, HIV infection has moved through networks of men injecting drugs and has spread to their wives. Other states have only just begun to detect HIV.

In China, HIV infection rates remain relatively low, with only about half a million people in a population of over a billion estimated to be HIV positive. The bulk of new infections were concentrated in drug injectors, and drug use by injection seems to be increasing. HIV prevalence in drug injectors in the densely populated coastal province of Guangdong rose from virtually nothing at the start of 1998 to 11 per cent by the start of 1999. Since over half of injectors reported sharing needles in behavioural surveys, HIV infection levels are likely to rise rapidly in the future. The potential for HIV to spread beyond China's drug-injecting population certainly exists. Massive population movements and increasing disparity in income have fuelled the sex industry in China. It is estimated that there may be as many as four million sex workers throughout the country. Behavioural surveys show that more than five out of 10 sex workers have never used a condom to protect themselves and their clients from STDs and HIV; in some areas the figure is nine out of 10.

Chart 3.4   The impact of rising condom use in Thailand[4]

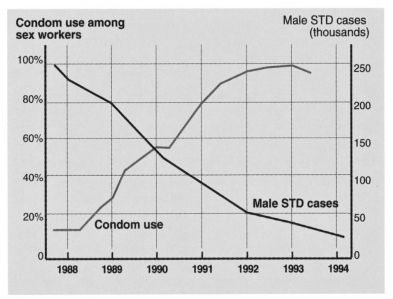

The country worthy of special mention is Thailand. This is one of the success stories of HIV prevention. In 1991, the Thai government stepped up its prevention efforts. One of the cornerstones was to make it compulsory for condoms to be used in brothels. The results were encouraging, as Chart 3.4 shows. As condom use rose, the incidence of STDs fell. It may also be that there was a significant change in sexual behaviour, for example fewer brothel visits, but this is rather harder to measure.

HIV surveillance is also beginning to show encouraging results. In the badly affected northern Thai province of Chiang Rai, the percentage of pregnant HIV-positive women fell from a peak of 6,4 per cent in 1994 to 4,6 per cent in 1997. This was particularly marked in younger women. In women under 25 experiencing their first pregnancy, HIV prevalence fell by 40 per cent over the same three-year period. The fall is remarkably consistent with a slightly earlier decline in HIV prevalence among young male military conscripts in northern Thailand.

Africa

The picture in Africa is also mixed. While North Africa is relatively free, sub-Saharan Africa is currently the epicentre of HIV and AIDS. At the beginning of 2000, it was estimated that 23,3 million people in sub-Saharan Africa have HIV or AIDS. This means that 70 per cent of the world's infections are found in an area with 10 per cent of the global population. About 90 per cent of infant and child infections are found here.

AIDS is the worst infectious disease to hit Africa in recorded history. According to the World Bank, 'deaths due to HIV/AIDS in Africa will soon surpass the 20 million Europeans killed by the plague epidemic of 1347-1351'.[5]

The statistics are frightening:
■ In the past decade, 12 million people in sub-Saharan Africa have died of AIDS – one-quarter being children.
■ Each day, AIDS claims another 5 500 men, women and children.
■ In 1998, AIDS was the largest killer, accounting for 1,8 million deaths in sub-Saharan Africa, nearly double the one million deaths from malaria and eight times the 209 000 deaths from TB.

44

■ A 15-year-old in Zambia has a 60 per cent chance of dying from AIDS.[6]

Population-based surveys show that infection levels in men are lower than in women in sub-Saharan Africa. On average, the 15 studies conducted in both rural and urban areas in nine different African countries suggest that between 12 and 13 African women are infected for every 10 African men. UNAIDS/WHO estimate that, at the end of 1999, 12,2 million women and 10,1 million men aged 15-49 were living with HIV in sub-Saharan Africa. This implies a future skewing of the demography of many African countries with men outnumbering women.

However, the epidemic is not uniform in Africa. In many West African countries, the spread of HIV seems to be slow and in some cases even contained. It is not clear whether this situation will continue. There is a significant epidemic emerging in Nigeria. But the worst situation is in the eastern and southern regions of Africa. In Uganda, the epidemic originally spread rapidly but now appears to have peaked. This has lessons for South Africa and we will return to it.

**Chart 3.5[7] HIV epidemics in developing countries
(i.e. chart excludes developed countries)**

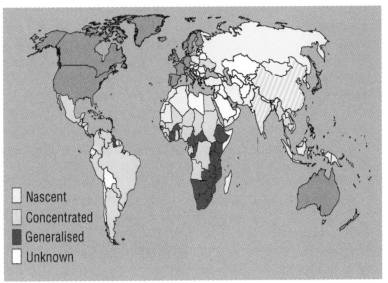

☐ Nascent
☐ Concentrated
■ Generalised
☐ Unknown

Another way of viewing the epidemics around the world has been put forward by the World Bank.[8]

They identify three stages of epidemic:

■ *Nascent:* HIV is less than five per cent in all known subpopulations presumed to practise high-risk behaviour.

■ *Concentrated:* HIV prevalence is above five per cent in *one or more* subpopulations presumed to practise high-risk behaviour; but among women attending urban antenatal clinics it is still below five per cent.

■ *Generalised.* HIV has spread far beyond the original subpopulations with high-risk behaviour, which are now heavily infected. Prevalence among women attending urban antenatal clinics is five per cent or more.

A breakdown on these lines is shown for the world in Chart 3.5 and for Africa in Chart 3.6. Unfortunately, all of southern Africa is experiencing a generalised epidemic.

Chart 3.6[9]   African HIV epidemics

4 The epidemic in South Africa

AIDS cases

The first two cases of AIDS were identified in South Africa in 1982. For the first eight years, the epidemic was primarily located among white homosexuals. Nonetheless, as the number of cases rose, so the disease began spreading among other groups. In July 1991, the number of heterosexually transmitted cases equalled the number of homosexual cases. Since then the homosexual epidemic has been completely overshadowed by the heterosexual epidemic. The steady increase in AIDS cases over the first eight years is shown in Chart 4.1, while the race and transmission categories are shown in Chart 4.2.

Chart 4.1   Annual AIDS case totals in South Africa[1]

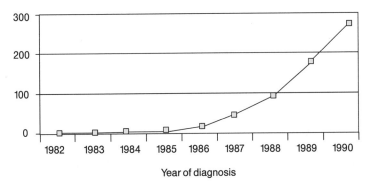

Year of diagnosis

MYTH
AIDS is a disease of gay white men in South Africa.
REALITY
Since 1991 there have been more heterosexuals infected than homosexuals, and the disease has spread among all race groups.

47

Chart 4.2   AIDS cases by race and transmission mechanism (up to 1990)[2]

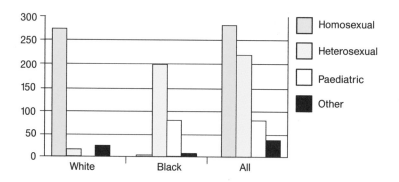

People working on AIDS in the 1980s felt it was inevitable that HIV would spread into the broader community. By 1991, the AIDS case data collected by the Department of National Health and Population Development showed that this was indeed the case. Over the next few years, the pattern of reported AIDS cases began to mirror that of all the countries in southern Africa. Chart 2.5 on page 32 shows the distribution of cases by age and gender in South Africa in 1995.

MYTH

AIDS is a disease of black people in South Africa.

REALITY

As we would expect, in terms of *absolute numbers,* there are many more black people infected than other race groups. But there is evidence that AIDS is spreading through all groups in South Africa and is breaching class barriers.

Collection and publication of AIDS case data ceased in 1995. AIDS was no longer a notifiable disease and the Department of Health felt that the AIDS case data had little value. Indeed, unless the data are collected regularly and comprehensively, this view is correct.

There is anecdotal evidence to suggest that the number of AIDS cases is rising steadily. Reports in the press and elsewhere provide additional proof of increasing AIDS cases and deaths. Here is a sample of press and other reports:

■ 30 per cent of paediatric admissions and 50 per cent of adult medical admissions at Gauteng hospitals were HIV-related in 1998.[3]

■ The 40 per cent increase in mortality rates at Natalspruit Hospital on the East Rand could be attributed to AIDS.[4]

■ In Gauteng hospitals, the proportion of adult medical in-patients with HIV-related conditions varied from 26 to 70 per cent.[5]

■ A total of 405 babies died before their first birthday in the Cape Town municipality in the year to June 1998, a 23 per cent increase on the previous year.[6]

■ A Port Elizabeth hospital is sending AIDS babies home to make way for children with illnesses that can be cured. Every day at the hospital at least two babies are diagnosed with AIDS. They are admitted only once and then restricted to outpatient care. The AIDS fatality rate of one a year seven years ago has increased over the past two years to up to two deaths a week.[7]

■ The number of burials and cremations in Durban has shown a sharp increase in the past few years, from 2 592 in 1993/94 to 8 983 in 1997/98.

■ In Johannesburg, 70 000 people were buried or cremated in 1999 compared to 15 000 in 1994.[8]

HIV

The spread of HIV across all South African communities was further confirmed when, in 1990, the first antenatal survey was carried out. This found that 0,8 per cent of women attending the state clinics were HIV positive. The survey was limited as it excluded the home-land areas[9] at the time. On the basis of this survey, it was estimated that there were between 74 000 and 120 000 HIV-infected people in South Africa in 1990.[10]

Since 1990, the antenatal surveys have been carried out annually and take place every October/November. After the installation of the new government in 1994, the entire country was covered by the surveys. These surveys provide the baseline information on which calculations of overall HIV prevalence and numbers of cases and deaths are based.

49

The steady increase in HIV prevalence in antenatal clinic attenders is shown below in Chart 4.3. From 0,8 per cent in 1990, the prevalence rate for South Africa as a whole reached 22,4 per cent in 1999. The data are collected by province, health region and age of women.

MYTH

HIV has spread so far that prevention efforts are irrelevant.
REALITY
Prevention efforts must remain a priority because:
1. Even in the worst affected areas where up to 35 per cent of the community are infected, at least 65 per cent are not. They can remain uninfected.
2. Each year a new generation becomes sexually active, and they can be educated to take precautionary measures.
3. In parts of South Africa, HIV prevalence is low.

HIV by province

There are significant variations in HIV prevalence rate by province. This is tabulated in Chart 4.3. KwaZulu-Natal has consistently had the highest levels of HIV infection although it appears to have reached a ceiling in the last two years at 32,5 per cent. In 1998, Mpumalanga had the second highest prevalence rate of 30 per cent but it dropped in 1999 to 27,3 per cent, putting the province in third place behind the Free State. The latter meanwhile increased from 22,8 per cent to 27,9 per cent. Overall, the 1999 data reveal an increase in six provinces, a decrease in two and the status quo in one.

As will be argued in Chapter 6, it would appear that the epidemic in Africa has a natural ceiling of around 30 per cent for the adult prevalence rate. The latest figures tend to confirm this, but provinces well below this ceiling are catching up. Hence, prevention programmes are vital to stop the increase continuing in those provinces, but also to bring down the rates in the two provinces which are close to the maximum. Unfortunately, the latest figures also give warning that provinces on the high side in HIV infection are going to have to deal with a large rise in AIDS cases in the near future as a matter of top priority.

Chart 4.3   Provincial breakdown of HIV prevalence rate in women attending antenatal clinics in South Africa (per cent)

Province	1990	1991	1992	1993	1994	1995	1996	1997	1998	1999
KZ-Natal	1,6	2,9	4,8	9,6	14,4	18,2	19,9	26,9	32,5	32,5
Free State	0,6	1,6	2,9	4,1	9,2	11,0	17,5	20,0	22,8	27,9
Mpumalanga					12,2	16,2	15,8	22,6	30,0	27,3
Gauteng					6,4	12,0	15,5	17,1	22,5	23,8
North-West					6,7	8,3	25,1	18,1	21,3	23,0
E. Cape					4,5	6,0	8,1	12,6	15,9	18,0
Northern					3,0	4,9	8,0	8,2	11,5	11,4
N. Cape					1,8	5,3	6,5	8,6	9,9	10,1
W. Cape					1,2	1,7	3,1	6,3	5,2	7,1
South Africa	0,8	1,4	2,4	4,3	7,6	10,4	14,2	17,0	22,8	22,4

The antenatal clinic data are also available by age, as is shown in Chart 4.4. While the most alarming thing from 1994 to 1998 was the rate of increase of infection in the youngest age groups, the decrease in 1999 gives rise to some optimism. The turnaround may indicate that prevention messages are beginning to get through and cause a change in behaviour among young women up to the age of 29. Equally, the government may have enhanced the status of this segment of the population successfully through its affirmative action programmes, so that they have the power to say no. Time will tell.

Chart 4.4   Breakdown by age of infection in women attending antenatal clinics

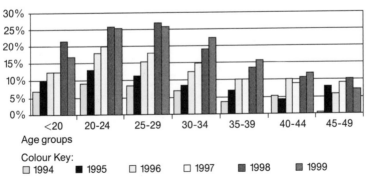

Age groups

Colour Key:
☐ 1994   ■ 1995   ☐ 1996   ☐ 1997   ■ 1998   ■ 1999

How representative are the data?

The HIV data shown above are for a very specific category of people – women attending the state antenatal clinics. This gives rise to two important questions:

■ To what extent can we view these data as representative of the broader situation in South Africa?

■ How can these data be used to project the epidemic into the future?

In a number of countries there have been population-based studies that have looked at the HIV prevalence in the broader population. These indicate that antenatal clinic data tend, if anything, to underestimate the HIV prevalence among sexually active women. As referred to in a previous chapter, the reason is that HIV infection reduces fertility over time. This means that women who have been infected for some time are less likely to fall pregnant and therefore will not be surveyed. However, the greater chance of infection among women means that there will be more women than men infected.

In order to estimate infections in the adult population, a ratio for female-to-male infections has to be established (and this may change over time). There is one HIV data set for a general population from Hlabisa district in KwaZulu-Natal which indicates that antenatal clinic data can be considered to be representative of the broader population. This is shown in Chart 4.5.

Chart 4.5   HIV prevalence in Hlabisa (1992-1997)[11]

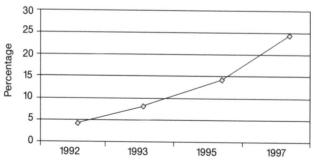

One important point about South Africa is that there does not appear to be much difference in the epidemic between urban and rural areas. This is not the case in African countries to the north, where rural areas generally have lower prevalence. South Africa's mobile population and good transport infrastructure mean that HIV has spread throughout the country.

Using proper statistical techniques, therefore, epidemiologists are fairly confident that they can take the antenatal clinic data and estimate HIV prevalence levels for each of the important groups in the South African population: adult females, adult males and children. These can then be turned into absolute numbers. The current calculation of the total number of infected South Africans in the past, present and future is shown in Chart 4.6.

Chart 4.6   Total number of HIV-infected South Africans

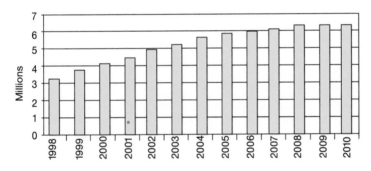

An analysis of the number of infections is shown in Chart 4.7. There are three estimates: low, best and high. It should be noted that even the highest estimated total is more conservative than the previous chart. Moreover, the recent advances in treatment mean that the number of babies infected by their mothers can be reduced with the appropriate interventions.

Projecting the epidemic

One of the real benefits of data is in helping people to look into the future. To do this, we can obviously build on the data that we have just presented on South Africa. But it is also instructive to look at the

Chart 4.7   Analysis of prevalence among HIV-infected South Africans (2000)[12]

	Females	Males	Babies	Total
Low estimate	1 870 000	1 358 000	129 000	3 357 000
Best estimate	1 957 000	1 412 000	132 000	3 501 000
High estimate	2 036 000	1 462 000	135 000	3 633 000

evidence from other countries in the region which may be more or less advanced in the HIV/AIDS cycle than we are.

UNAIDS makes estimates of the adult prevalence rate, the number of people living with HIV/AIDS and the number of orphans. These figures are available by country from the UNAIDS website *www.unaids.org*. A comparison of South Africa's neighbours is shown in Chart 4.8. It highlights the fact that, although the data are rather old, there are a number of countries that have significantly higher rates of infection than South Africa. Again this is important because it stresses the need for effective prevention. *We can turn the epidemic round; we do have some time.*

Chart 4.8   UNAIDS estimates for southern Africa in 1998[13]

Country	Adult prevalence rate (per cent)	Number of adults & children living with HIV/AIDS	Estimated number of orphans
Botswana	25,1	190 000	25 000
Lesotho	8,4	85 000	8 500
Mozambique	14,2	1 200 000	150 000
Namibia	19,9	150 000	7 300
South Africa	12,9	2 900 000	180 000
Swaziland	18,5	84 000	7 200
Zambia	19,1	770 000	360 000
Zimbabwe	25,8	1 500 000	360 000
Total/average	Av. 12	10 805 000	2 214 000

Note: Orphans are defined as children under the age of 15 who have lost their mother or their mother and father.

The epidemic seems to have a natural peak if one considers the data from Botswana, the country that is experiencing one of the worst HIV epidemics in the world. In Chart 4.9, it is noticeable that the

HIV prevalence rose to just over 40 per cent in Francistown in 1996, but has not risen further.

Chart 4.9   HIV prevalence (per cent) in selected locations in Botswana (antenatal clinic attenders)

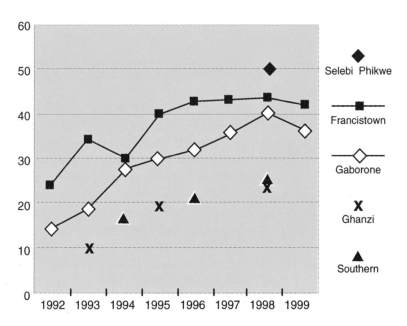

MYTH
Most of the population will inevitably be infected.
REALITY
As with all diseases, there appears to be a natural peak in HIV. Some people will not be at risk; some will be lucky; some will change their behaviour as they see others dying around them. Thus, the adult HIV prevalence rate is unlikely to exceed 30 per cent in South Africa, although some segments of the population and some regions will experience higher rates of infection.

In order to assess the likely social and economic impact of HIV/AIDS, we need an idea of the future course of the epidemic and hence how many people will fall ill and die. Mathematical models (which are translated into computer programmes) may be used to create projections of the future course of the epidemic and the consequent impacts, and more specifically, estimate the magnitude of these impacts. There are several different types of models in use and several software packages available for projecting the HIV/AIDS epidemic. These range from the very simplistic to the highly complex.

MYTH
The future course of the HIV epidemic is inevitable and we have to watch helplessly as it unfolds.
REALITY
Most projections show what will happen to HIV prevalence if interventions are not put in place and do not work. The whole purpose of this book is to encourage a variety of interventions which will curb the spread of the epidemic in the long run. However, even with successful and sustainable preventive measures, we can be fairly sure of the number of adult AIDS cases and deaths over the next four to seven years because these people are already infected. We can also predict the number of orphans. The only development which will upset all forecasts in the short run is the provision of cheap, effective treatment which extends the lives of people living with HIV indefinitely. This remains a wild card – possible but unlikely. A vaccine/cure is further off.

HIV/AIDS projection models may be used for several different purposes, such as:
■ projecting HIV prevalence rates and numbers;
■ projecting future numbers of AIDS cases, AIDS-related deaths and orphans by year;
■ examining the demographic impact of AIDS and addressing questions regarding the impact of AIDS on population growth rates, the population age structure, numbers of orphans,[14] and life expectancy;
■ simulating different intervention strategies and comparing their strengths and weaknesses;

■ assessing the impact of the AIDS epidemic, for example how it will increase health expenditure and interact with other diseases such as tuberculosis; and

■ creating different scenarios which illustrate the effect of different assumptions on the projected outcome.

In order to use models to create projections of the future course of the HIV/AIDS epidemic and its likely impact, we need reliable information about what the current situation is. All models depend on data. However, the amount and type of input data required will depend on the type of model being used and the questions to be answered. South Africa has two locally developed models, that of Peter Doyle and colleagues of Metropolitan Life; and the Actuarial Society of Southern Africa model which can be found at *www. assa.co.za* .

In September 1998, the Department of Health organised a meeting of experts to develop a consensus on the status, future spread and impact of HIV/AIDS in South Africa. This brought together epidemiologists, actuaries, economists, health specialists and others with an interest in the issue, and resulted in an agreed set of projections.[15]

In addition, there are some public domain models that have been developed outside South Africa, the most accessible being the *Spectrum* package of models.[16] It is important to keep in mind that models are simply tools which may be used to guide decision making. Models are, by definition, a *representation* of an *aspect* of reality and they cannot possibly replicate the complexity that the real situation presents. Furthermore, the degree to which the outputs of models are applicable to the real world depends upon the nature of the model itself, and the reliability and validity of the data that are used. When using models, it is important to bear in mind what the model was designed for and what the limitations are.

Given these closing comments, we will address the future course of the epidemic in South Africa and its demographic impact in Chapter 6.

5 The severity of South Africa's epidemic

Before contemplating the future, we must answer two crucial questions. Firstly, why has HIV spread so rapidly in South Africa; and secondly, why will the impact be so severe? South Africa has experienced one of the fastest growth rates of the epidemic in the world.

In order to understand the dynamics of the epidemic, it is necessary to appreciate that South African society is both particularly susceptible to the spread of HIV and particularly vulnerable to its impact.

MYTH
I can be cured of AIDS if I sleep with a virgin.
REALITY
This is an urban legend doing the rounds in South Africa which illustrates just how desperate the epidemic has made people feel.

Susceptibility is defined as the chance of an individual becoming infected. The extent of susceptibility will be determined by the riskiness of the environment in which the individual lives and works. Factors at play may be environmental, infrastructural, cultural, economic or social. Vulnerability describes those features of a society that make it more or less likely that the increased adult illness and death will adversely affect it or segments of it.

South Africa, as a nation, is highly susceptible to the spread of HIV and vulnerable to the impact of AIDS, but there are segments in the society which are particularly susceptible and vulnerable. In South Africa, the highest rates of infection are amongst people between 20 and 44 years old. Because a sizeable percentage of South Africa's population is aged between these years, AIDS has the potential to have a devastating effect on social, economic, and, above all, human development. It will take time for the economic and social impacts to be felt, but demographic impact is already being seen, as will be described in the next chapter.

The reasons for the rapid spread

Despite a relatively late start, HIV has taken off in South Africa. The apartheid system may have delayed the onset of the epidemic, but its legacy is a fertile environment for HIV's rapid spread.

Given that the main mode of transmission of HIV is sex, it would seem reasonable that the virus is spreading so quickly in South Africa because of the level of sexual activity, the type of sex or the range of partners. However, no statistics are available to support this point of view. Indeed, one study that has been done to compare sexual behaviour in different countries comes to the conclusion that South Africa is pretty normal by world standards.

The Durex Global Sex Survey carried out in 1996, 1997 and 1998 included South Africa in 1998 for the first time. In 1998, the survey covered 14 countries and a total of 10 000 respondents. While it may not be academically rigorous, the biases and 'lie factors' are probably consistent across the nations sampled. The highlights are shown in Chart 5.1.[1]

Chart 5.1   Sexual behaviours in selected countries

Country	Age at first sexual experience	Average number of episodes of sexual intercourse per annum
USA	16,3	138
Britain	16,7	112
Australia	17,1	112
Thailand	19,6	80
Germany	17,4	112
South Africa	17,3	109

Intuitively, some readers might feel that the first figure for South Africa is on the high side[2] and the second on the low side. Yet, even if one were to adjust the figures accordingly, it would not alter the conclusion of the survey that South Africans seem to be no more nor less sexually active than their foreign counterparts. This means that we have to look for other factors that are driving the epidemic. Crucial ones are the level of other STDs besides HIV; sexual mixing patterns; and the number of concurrent partners.

There are plenty of data to show that South Africans, especially the poorer ones, have higher levels of STDs than the citizens of the other countries listed in Chart 5.1. Moreover, many of the STD cases in South Africa never get treated. More than 50 per cent of antenatal clinic attendees have been found to be infected with at least one STD.[3] Up to 15 per cent are seropositive for syphilis, compared to three per cent in Botswana.[4]

Sexual mixing patterns are about the number and type of people with whom an individual has sex. In most societies, the circle of partners is usually quite small. The broader it is, the more possible it is for a virus like HIV to spread. In South Africa, as will be expanded on later in this chapter, the social upheavals of modern times have raised considerably the potential number of sexual partners that the average person is expected to have during his or her lifetime. The third factor of concurrent partnerships greatly assists the spread of HIV. Thus, the man who has a simultaneous sexual relationship with several women is more likely to transmit the virus (or have the virus transmitted to him) than the man who practises serial monogamy, i.e. regularly changes partners but is faithful to one at a time. A mobile society like South Africa, particularly along the main transport arteries, offers great scope for concurrent partners.

MYTH

African society has always been promiscuous, and this is the driving force behind the AIDS epidemic in South Africa.

REALITY

As in the West, sexual patterns have changed as a result of a multiplicity of factors. In South Africa, social upheaval rather than sexual liberation may have been responsible for an increase in the numbers of sexual partners. But there is no evidence to prove this.

Survey of sexual behaviour

Most of the previous section is hypothesis in the absence of hard facts. It does seem preposterous that we have so little pertinent data about a virus that is such a threat to our society. But then it is related to sex and people do not like talking openly about sex. Taboos and prejudices mar any debate on the matter. As mentioned in Chapter 2, the only way we will get a decent lock on the problem is to have better data. However difficult it is to undertake, we would recommend a proper survey of sexual behaviour in South Africa so that we can identify where the points of leverage are in formulating strategies to stop the spread of HIV. In America, if an equivalent proportion of Americans were HIV positive (30 million), there is no doubt that a multitude of academic and governmental surveys would have been done to establish more precisely the sexual and social mechanisms through which the virus spreads.

A theoretical framework

Nevertheless, one must start somewhere and the rest of this chapter is devoted to a conceptual framework developed by Barnett and Whiteside[5] to explain the severity of the epidemic in South Africa. They argue that the shape of an epidemic curve, i.e. how many people are infected and how rapidly the epidemic spreads, will be determined by two key variables:
- The degree of social cohesion in society; and
- The overall level of wealth.

Social cohesion is a concept that needs further explanation. It is partially derived from civil society, that part of society which occupies the space between the individual and the state and the degree to which there are perceived and acted-on community interests. Civil society includes voluntary organisations, nongovernmental organisations, parent-teacher associations, and indeed any grouping of people outside the household and workplace. However, social cohesion is also derived from a nation's political and cultural systems: whether they are inclusive or divisive. Wealth is simply the level of income per head and needs no further explanation. Income inequality is taken into account, since societies with low social cohesion and high wealth invariably have high Gini indexes, indicating great inequality.[6]

The argument is simple: societies with high levels of social cohesion and high incomes will not experience a serious epidemic (the US, UK and France); those with high levels of social cohesion and low incomes will see only a slow-growing epidemic (Senegal and North African countries); those with low levels of social cohesion and low incomes will have severe epidemics but they take time to develop (Uganda and Rwanda). It is countries with low levels of social cohesion and relatively high incomes that face the most rapidly growing epidemics and highest levels of infection. Unfortunately, South Africa falls into the last category, as Chart 5.2 indicates.

In applying this conceptual framework to South Africa, one can explain why the epidemic has been so severe to date; why it is located where it is; and what may happen.

Chart 5.2 Comparative income, equity, urbanisation and mobility

Country	Per capita income (1998$)	Gini index	Urbanisation (per cent)	Number of vehicles per 1 000 people
Botswana	3 600	–	68	44
South Africa	2 880	58	50	142
Uganda	320	41	13	4
Kenya	330	58	31	13
Zambia	330	46	44	26
Tanzania	210	38	26	5
Zimbabwe	610	57	31	32
Senegal	530	54	45	14

Under the apartheid system, the country was subjected to extreme social engineering, designed for the benefit of the minority white population. The state sought to control who could live and work where. Government policy stated: 'Bantu are only temporarily resident in European areas for as long as they offer their labour there. As soon as they become, for some reason or other, no longer fit for work or superfluous in the labour market they are expected to return to their country of origin.'[7] The 'country of origin' included both the homelands and the neighbouring independent countries.

South Africa's black population was forced into crowded, impoverished homelands which led to the breakdown of traditional cultural structures. Adults, mainly men, migrated to the urban areas to work in white-owned factories and mines and to live in single-sex hostels. They were prevented by law from bringing their families. This created a culture of urban and rural wives and prostitution – not necessarily for cash but as part of a survival strategy. Many children were cared for by adults other than their parents; and, in the wake of family break-ups, child abuse and child prostitution became a new phenomenon. Health services were limited, which meant many diseases including STDs went untreated.

At the peak in 1985, there were 1 833 636 South Africans working as migrants. This meant that they were not regarded as resident in the areas where they worked. Of these, 771 397 came from the 'independent' homelands of Transkei, Bophuthatswana, Venda and Ciskei; and 1 062 239 from the 'self-governing' homelands of Lebowa, Gazankulu, Qwa Qwa, KwaZulu, KwaNdebele and KaNgwane. In addition, there were 27 814 Batswana, 139 827 Basotho, 30 144 Malawians, 68 665 Mozambicans and 22 255 Swazi employed officially as migrants in South Africa.[8] Equally, one must not overlook many illegal migrants, mainly employed in the agricultural sector.

Although there are now fewer migrants and South Africans can live where they choose, the legacy of apartheid remains. In some industries, particularly mining, employment conditions have improved considerably and a greater proportion of the labour force is drawn from local residents living in the neighbourhood of the mines. Nonetheless, migration is a way of life for many workers and the mines still provide hostel accommodation for them. Of course, it must be acknowledged that for foreign workers and their governments the ending of the migrant labour system would be a mixed blessing. Although the numbers are declining, migration remains an important source of employment for tens of thousands southern Africans, as is shown in Chart 5.3. Remittances from the migrants are an important source of income for many dependants and a critical source of foreign exchange for the governments concerned.

Chart 5.3   Trends in employment of foreign migrants in the South African mining industry[9]

Country of origin	1984	1989	1994	1998
Lesotho	75 787	98 085	84 700	60 450
Botswana	18 599	15 229	10 837	7 752
Swaziland	12 152	16 555	14 829	10 336
Mozambique	42 294	44 015	44 044	51 913

Suffice it to say, the pattern of men moving away from their families for long periods, living in crowded and alien conditions with little power over their lives, created the ideal situation for the spread of all STDs.

Inequality

In 1993 in South Africa, the richest 10 per cent of the population received 47,3 per cent of the income; whereas the poorest 40 per cent of the people had only a 9,1 per cent share. Land inequalities meant that 71 per cent of the rural population – mainly black – lived on 14 per cent of the land, while the balance of farmland was owned by only 67 000 farmers, almost all white. Inequality assisted (and continues to assist) in the spread of HIV because poor women had few financial resources and were forced into sexual relationships to ensure the survival of themselves and their children.

Legislation and formalisation of discrimination

The education of black people was circumscribed. They were prevented by law from doing certain jobs in white areas. Government even sought to regulate sexual behaviour, and the notorious Immorality Act prohibited sexual intercourse between the different race groups. All this combined to create a widespread philosophy of fatalism – a perception that 'what will be, will be' – which in turn diminished individual worth, responsibility and accountability. This feeling is still prevalent and makes people live for today without valuing tomorrow. It can be summed up in a shrug of the shoulders and the response: 'If AIDS kills me in five years' time, so what?'

Conflict

The apartheid system could not last. But, during its final years, the cycle of oppression and resistance led to the almost total disruption of civil society. The slogan 'make the townships ungovernable' was to have far-reaching consequences. In addition, there was a militarisation of the society. Armed forces included the defence force, homeland armies, liberation movements, self-defence units and political militias. Apart from the internal conflict, there were wars being fought in Angola and Namibia. Conflict between the armed wings of the political parties continued up to the 1994 election, and in KwaZulu-Natal continues still, albeit at a much lower level.

It is well known that military forces have higher levels of infection than the general population; refugees are particularly susceptible to HIV; and conflict results in the inability to absorb and act on messages contained in educational programmes on HIV. The subject has little immediacy to those involved. All this may go some way to explaining the fact that KwaZulu-Natal has the highest level of HIV in South Africa.

Indeed, one astonishing fact that emerged from the Truth and Reconciliation Commission was the use of HIV as a weapon. According to submissions made by two apartheid-era security officers, Willie Nortjé and Andries van Heerden, at the TRC in 1999, askaris (former ANC operatives who had gone over to work for the apartheid state security forces) were used to spread the disease. Ones known to be HIV positive were employed at two Hillbrow hotels, the Chelsea and Little Rose, in 1990, with the explicit instruction to infect sex workers.[10]

The ending of apartheid, and in 1994 the election of the new government, resulted in the relaxation of the draconian controls on society. But they were not immediately replaced by a strong civil society – hardly surprising, as this is something that has to be built over time rather than imposed. In addition, there was no immediate redistribution of resources or a lessening of income inequality.

Crime and rape

Crime and gang violence are now the main source of conflict in South Africa. As a consequence, rape and gang rape have become extremely potent methods of spreading HIV. In 1998, 49 280 rapes and 4 851 sexual assaults were reported. When the 179 incest reports are added to these figures, a total of 54 310 sexual crimes were officially recorded in that year. However, the definition of rape is narrow; and, as a crime, it is seriously underreported. Information revealed by a study conducted by the Institute of Security Studies found that in only 29 per cent of cases did women tell *anyone* (and not usually the police) of their experiences of violence, and as many as 41 per cent had never told anyone at all.[11] If this is

65

the situation within metropolitan areas, the rate of reporting is likely to be even lower in rural areas. Rape Crisis in Cape Town estimates that the actual figure for sexual crimes could be over one million per annum on the basis that only one in twenty cases is reported.[12]

Obviously, rape has associated with it much higher odds of HIV transmission because the victim is more likely to bleed as a result of being forcibly violated. There is every reason to assume that the HIV prevalence rate among rapists is just as high as, if not higher than, the average adult prevalence rate. Rape therefore brings the possibility of premature illness and death for the victims.

Another scary scenario is that, as more young men are informed of their HIV status, they will become more reckless in their sexual forays as they compensate for not having long to live.

The severe impact in South Africa

As a result of the growth in HIV prevalence, and the failure to control the spread of HIV, South Africa faces a major AIDS epidemic. Instead of being able to focus purely, or even largely, on prevention activities, the country is about to have to deal with the consequences of large-scale conversion from HIV to AIDS. These will be far-reaching.

In terms of impact, there is a great deal that is unknown. Nowhere in the world has the epidemic run its course, and it will be many years before it does. AIDS is a disaster, but: 'Disasters do not happen, they unfold'.[13] The implication is that, in theory, it should be possible to take the model of the future course of the epidemic, plan for its impact, and consider it in national and regional policy.

The effect of AIDS on South Africa will be covered in the next chapters. However, at this point it is important to note that the effect will be serious and will probably be more so than in most other countries. There are a number of reasons for this.

Most obviously, the scale of the epidemic in South Africa is considerable. The 1999 data show that 22,4 per cent of antenatal clinic attenders are infected. Although this percentage is a shade below the previous year's, it could well rise further before the epidemic is brought under control. As the epidemic progresses, the sheer number of illnesses, deaths and orphans will be greater in South Africa than in other countries.

The fact that South Africa has a more developed economy may magnify the impact. There will be two mechanisms at work. Firstly, South Africa is more dependent on skilled labour than other countries in the region, and the skills base is extremely small. Losses of skilled and professional staff could hamper business and government operations, and possibly slow economic growth. The second mechanism is that South Africans have more interaction with and expectation of service from their government than is the case in the rest of Africa. Examples are:

■ Pensions – there is only one other country where the elderly can expect to be paid a pension and that is Botswana which has a pension of P117 or R154. In South Africa a pensioner can expect to receive R520 per month.

■ Health care – all South Africans are entitled to health care and, in the case of pregnant mothers and children under the age of six, this is free.

■ Provision of housing and basic utilities such as water and electricity is a national priority and delivery of these is being achieved, albeit more slowly than originally envisaged.

■ There is a grant for foster children. This is paid following a successful application to the court by a nonrelated person to have a child placed in his or her care. The payment is R350 per month. In practice the grant has been paid to family members, particularly to grandparents.

This means that the expectations of assistance and health care as the epidemic develops will be greater. Concurrently, the human resources that are expected to provide these services will, in turn, be depleted by the epidemic. Just as the government and other principal role players are trying to construct a civil society, the country will be waging an uncivil war against an invisible enemy more ruthless than any human adversary. It poses an enormous challenge.

6 Projections and demographic impact

In order to understand and plan for the impact of AIDS, we need to know how many people are and will be infected; when they will fall ill; what care they will need (and get); when they will die; and how many children they will leave behind. Ideally, we also need to know who they are in terms of income, education and skills, employment and location. As is apparent, our available data fall far short of this. Furthermore, some of the data that would be valuable for planning purposes is confidential and obtaining it would infringe individual rights. Despite these drawbacks, it is still possible to estimate the

Chart 6.1   Basic HIV/AIDS projection 1997-2010

	1997	1998	1999	2000	2001	2002	2003
Adult HIV prevalence rate (per cent)	8,9	10,7	12,4	14,0	15,3	16,5	17,6
HIV prevalence (000's)							
– adults	2 128	2 598	3 053	3 475	3 871	4 235	4 577
– children	87	114	144	173	201	226	250
– total	2 215	2 712	3 197	3 648	4 072	4 461	4 827
AIDS cases (000's)							
– adults	57	83	118	161	213	272	336
– children	18	25	33	42	50	59	67
– total	75	108	151	203	263	331	403
AIDS deaths (000's)							
– adults	47	67	93	125	161	203	246
– children	14	19	25	31	36	42	47
– total	61	86	118	156	197	245	293
Orphans	60	96	147	217	309	425	568

Note: Adult denotes a person 15 to 59 years old; children are 0 to 14 years old; and

current position and project the epidemic into the future. It should be remembered that current AIDS deaths are due to HIV infections over the past eight or so years. Current HIV infections will result in deaths over the next 10 years.

Projecting the epidemic in South Africa

In 1998, as part of a paper for the United Nations Development Programme, projections were commissioned from Metropolitan Life by one of the authors. These are shown in Chart 6.1.[1]

Several points must be made concerning this projection:
■ We are already running ahead of schedule because the latest estimate for 2000 is about 4,2 million HIV-positive adults and children compared to the figure in the table of 3,6 million. South Africa was only expected to reach 4,2 million in 2002;

	2004	2005	2006	2007	2008	2009	2010
Adult HIV prevalence rate (per cent)	18,6	19,5	20,2	20,7	21,1	21,4	21,7
HIV prevalence (000's)							
– adult	4 887	5 161	5 387	5 555	5 675	5 764	5 830
– children	271	291	309	326	342	354	365
– total	5 158	5 452	5 696	5 881	6 017	6 118	6 195
AIDS cases (000's)							
– adult	403	469	532	588	635	674	705
– children	74	81	88	93	99	104	108
– total	477	550	620	681	734	778	813
AIDS deaths (000's)							
– adult	291	334	373	408	437	460	478
– children	52	56	60	64	68	71	73
– total	343	390	433	472	505	531	551
Orphans	734	921	1 123	1 333	1 543	1 746	1 936

orphans are children up to 14 years old who lost their mother due to AIDS.

69

■ The numbers of AIDS cases and AIDS deaths lag significantly behind the numbers of HIV-positive people, but rise inexorably;

■ Although the number of HIV-positive people flattens out towards the end of the projection at just over six million, incidence is still high but is being offset by the rising number of AIDS deaths;

■ In this model, the adult prevalence rate rises to just under 22 per cent in 2010. In light of experience elsewhere in Africa, the final ceiling for the adult prevalence rate can be as high as 30 per cent. This would imply an eventual total of about eight million people infected, nearly double the present figure;

■ The number of orphans in South Africa is forecast to reach close to two million by 2010.

The impact of HIV on mortality is very clearly illustrated in Chart 6.2. This shows the steady and inevitable rise in the number of deaths from AIDS. By about 2006, there will be as many deaths from AIDS as from all other causes. It should be remembered that AIDS mainly kills young adults in the economically active age group.

Chart 6.2   Normal deaths, AIDS deaths and new HIV infections[2]

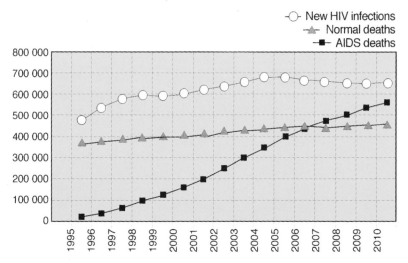

70

KwaZulu-Natal (KZN): a case study[3]

Projections can also be done for provinces or districts. In 1999, projections were commissioned for KZN. Chart 6.3 shows that the adult HIV prevalence rate is expected to rise until 2006 when it will peak at 29 per cent. Nevertheless, *it should be noted that the future of the epidemic can be influenced through successful interventions*; the curve could peak sooner and lower; and it could be made to fall faster.

Chart 6.3   Projected total and adult HIV prevalence rates in KZN[4]

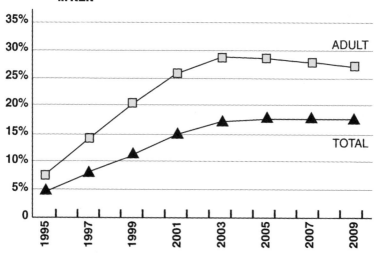

—☐— Adult population HIV % (15-59)
—▲— Total population HIV %

If the percentages are translated into figures, then an estimated 1 115 000 adults in KZN are infected already. There are about 71 000 people living with AIDS and in 2000 there will be an estimated 53 500 deaths. The projected deaths are shown in Chart 6.4 while the projected number of orphans is shown in Chart 6.5. While we have stressed that new infections can be prevented, many of these deaths and most of the orphans are inevitable as they are a consequence of infections that have already taken place. This is an impact that must be planned for, although treatments are being developed and some may be affordable in the KZN context.

Chart 6.4   Projected AIDS deaths in KZN[5]

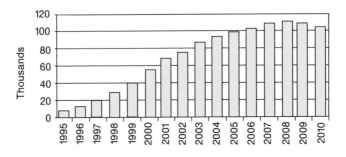

Chart 6.5   Projected AIDS orphans in KZN[6]

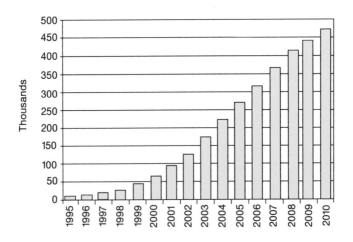

One of the conclusions of the study is that the total population of KZN will continue to grow up to 2008, after which it is expected to register a small decline in numbers (see chart 6.6). In 2010, there will be 9 095 000 people in the province, compared to a figure in the absence of AIDS of 10 723 000. Currently, there are 8 870 000. These numbers are important because they indicate that, under all scenarios, the enormous backlog in housing, health and education will continue to be a problem. Nevertheless, the population structure is changing and growth is slowing – factors which must be built into planning.

Chart 6.6 Population projections for KZN (000's)

Year	Without AIDS	With AIDS	% difference
1996	8 394	8 394	0
1997	8 557	8 532	0,3
1998	8 730	8 660	0,8
1999	8 903	8 774	1,5
2000	9 076	8 870	2,3
2001	9 250	8 946	3,4
2002	9 412	9 005	4,3
2003	9 586	9 047	5,6
2004	9 759	9 076	7,0
2005	9 921	9 092	8,4
2006	10 084	9 099	9,8
2007	10 246	9 101	11,2
2008	10 409	9 099	12,6
2009	10 560	9 097	13,9
2010	10 723	9 095	15,2

Demographic impact[7]

AIDS is a demographic issue because it affects the major demographic processes of mortality and fertility. The direct effects on mortality arise from the deaths of adults and children. The effects on fertility are indirect and less well understood. The accumulation of mortality and fertility effects leads to changes in the other demographic indicators like population growth and size.

Mortality

The most direct demographic consequence of AIDS is an increase in mortality. Without effective treatment of HIV infection, people develop AIDS and die. However, as we have already mentioned, recent advances in drug therapy have raised the hope that HIV infection may be controlled for some individuals. Progression to AIDS and death may be delayed or even averted. The high cost of the drugs and the difficulty in administering them are obstacles that still need to be overcome.

The age at which the majority of people are infected means AIDS increases mortality among those that typically have the lowest

73

Chart 6.7   Mortality rate by age with and without AIDS: 1997

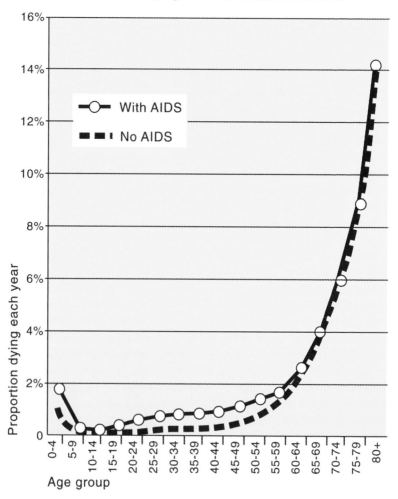

mortality rates. AIDS has been identified as the major cause of deaths of adults aged 15 to 44 in Abidjan and of adults aged 15 to 59 in Tanzania.[8] There are no data available on AIDS as a cause of death in South Africa yet. However, it can be modelled. Charts 6.7 and 6.8 show the impact of AIDS on age-specific mortality rates in 1997 and the projected impact for 2010, using the 1997 antenatal clinic prevalence data.

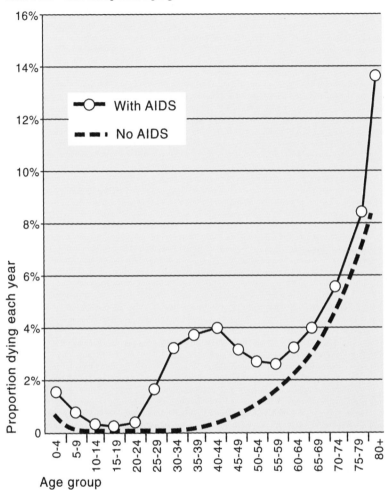

Chart 6.8   Mortality rate by age with and without AIDS: 2010

Legend:
- ─○─ With AIDS
- ▪ ▪ ▪ No AIDS

Y-axis: Proportion dying each year (0 to 16%)
X-axis: Age group (0-4, 5-9, 10-14, 15-19, 20-24, 25-29, 30-34, 35-39, 40-44, 45-49, 50-54, 55-59, 60-64, 65-69, 70-74, 75-79, 80+)

Infant and child mortality

An HIV-positive woman may pass the infection to the foetus during pregnancy or to the newborn child during delivery or through breast-feeding. Between 13 and 45 per cent of children born to infected mothers will be infected.[9] The percentage will vary with the stage of the epidemic, availability of antenatal care, and general health of the infected women. Most HIV children develop AIDS and die within a few years of birth, increasing infant and child mortality. Countries which have shown the greatest gains in improving infant and child mortality indicators are likely to see the greatest reversals, as is shown in Chart 6.9.[10]

Chart 6.9   Child mortality 1998 and 2010 with and without AIDS (rate per 1 000)

Country	1998		2010	
	With AIDS	Without AIDS	With AIDS	Without AIDS
Botswana	121	57	120	38
South Africa	96	70	100	49
Swaziland	103	84	152	78
Zimbabwe	123	51	116	32

Life expectancy

Life expectancy at birth is particularly sensitive to AIDS. Deaths of children and young adults mean a large number of years of life are lost. There are two main sources of information on this: the United Nations Development Programme, which has taken AIDS into account in its Human Development Reports since 1997; and the US Bureau of the Census, which has projected the impact of AIDS on current and future levels of life expectancy. It should be noted that all estimates of impact on life expectancy are modelled and not observed.

Chart 6.10 shows the effect of AIDS on life expectancy for selected southern African countries, as supplied by the UNDP. As well as life expectancy, the chart also shows the impact on the country's ranking according to the Human Development Index (HDI). The HDI was developed by the UNDP in 1990 to capture the concept that human development is about more than per capita income. It is discussed at greater length in the next chapter.

The US Bureau of the Census estimates of changes in life expectancy are shown in Chart 6.11 The differences between the two sets of data are because the UNDP has taken a rather more conservative view than the US Bureau.

Chart 6.10   UNDP life expectancy and ranking in the human development index[11]

	1996		1997		1998		1999	
	Life expect-ancy (years)	HDI rank	Life expect-ancy (years)	HDI rank	Life expect-ancy (years)	HDI rank	Life expect-ancy (years)	HDI rank
Botswana	65	71	52	97	52	97	47	122
South Africa	63	100	64	90	64	89	55	101
Swaziland	58	110	58	114	59	115	60	113
Namibia	59	116	56	118	56	107	52	115
Zimbabwe	53	124	49	129	49	130	44	130
Kenya	56	128	54	134	54	137	52	136
Zambia	49	136	43	143	43	146	40	151
Malawi	46	157	41	161	41	161	39	159

Chart 6.11   US Bureau of the Census – estimates of life expectancy (years)

	Botswana	South Africa	Swaziland	Zimbabwe
1998	40	56	39	39
2010	38	48	37	39

Fertility[12]

The effect on fertility will be threefold. Firstly, the number of births may be reduced if women die before reaching the end of their child-bearing years. The second effect is that HIV infection and AIDS reduce fertility through physiological means. Finally, AIDS aware-ness, the use of condoms and increased empowerment of women will reduce fertility. As the total fertility rate is already declining in South Africa on account of urbanisation and rising affluence, the epidemic and the programmes to fight it could cause the rate of descent to be steeper still.

Population size and growth

It is generally believed that the epidemic is unlikely to lead to negative population growth and an absolute decrease in population numbers. Obviously, there will be local exceptions where there is a combination of very high levels of HIV prevalence and rapidly

77

declining fertility, such as in parts of Zambia, Botswana, Zimbabwe and – in our case – KwaZulu-Natal. The US Bureau of the Census projections for South Africa are that in 1998 the annual population growth rate with AIDS was 1,4 per cent and without AIDS would have been 1,9 per cent. For 2010, the respective figures are 0,4 per cent with AIDS and 1,4 per cent without AIDS. Interestingly, very little research has yet been done to quantify the gender imbalance that is likely to ensue from the epidemic, with men outnumbering women.

MYTH
1. AIDS will cause national populations to fall.
2. The population of KZN is already declining.
REALITY
1. Even in the worst affected countries, it is unlikely that overall population growth rates will become sharply negative. What we will see is a slower growth rate and thus, in the years ahead, the population will be smaller than it would have been in the absence of AIDS. In South Africa, for example, it is estimated that without AIDS the population would have risen to 51,3 million in 2010. With AIDS it is now expected to reach 47 million.
2. Within the hardest hit regions in badly affected countries, the population could actually decline. In this regard, the population of KZN is projected to register a small drop after 2008.

It should be noted, however, that demographers have been very slow to consider AIDS as an issue. In our opinion the effects of increased mortality, change in fertility and behaviour may have a larger impact than currently predicted.

Dependency ratio

The dependency ratio is the number of dependants (usually children under the age of 15 and adults over the age of 64) per 100 adults of productive age, i.e. 15 to 64 years old. The increase in young adult deaths will be roughly balanced by the increase in child deaths, with the result that the dependency ratio does not change dramatically in the presence of an AIDS epidemic.[13] However, the dependency situation is adversely affected in other ways. AIDS increases the number of widows and widowers.[14] When parents die, children are often left in the care of grandparents or other members of the extended family or community. Grandparents themselves have no one to look after them anymore. Charts 6.12 and 6.13 reveal just how much AIDS will change the shape of the population.

Chart 6.12   Population pyramid for South Africa in 1998[15]

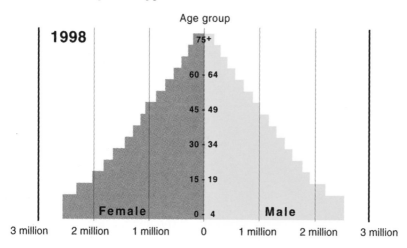

Chart 6.13   Population pyramid for South Africa in 2010[16]

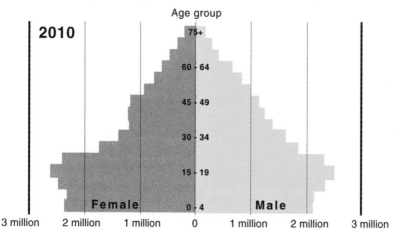

Orphans

South Africa currently has a high proportion of children who are not continuously cared for by either parent, and very high rates of care by aunts and by grandmothers. This is due to the history of displacement of people to implement the racially segregated society envisaged during the years of apartheid, combined with the migrant labour system. The epidemic inserts itself into this already fragile family environment, and one of its worst consequences is the creation of AIDS orphans. At present, South Africa is witnessing the emergence of child-headed households and the conversion of facilities designed for early childhood education into de facto residential homes. It has been estimated that KwaZulu-Natal will face 65 500 AIDS orphans by 2000 and nearly 500 000 by the year 2010.[17]

One of the major issues of the epidemic is the increase in orphaning. A problem arises with the definition of an orphan. UNAIDS defines an orphan as a child below the age of 15 who has lost either their mother or both their mother and father. However, this is very narrow because:

■ A child will begin to have needs that the family cannot meet and stresses that the family cannot alleviate when the parent falls ill and household income drops. Effectively 'orphaning' begins prior to the death of the parent.

■ Children may be 'orphaned' more than once – the first time when their parents die and then again if their grandparents (who are often the people who inherit the task of caring for the children) die.

■ Children who lose their fathers may lose financial resources which would have assisted them in their education, etc.

■ Reaching the age of 15 does not imply that orphans no longer have needs; indeed, they may be slower to mature.

Work done in other parts of Africa suggests that there may be up to three times as many children in need as are orphaned.

HIV/AIDS and national population projections

In order for the epidemic to be considered in the nation's population policy there are two preconditions:

■ Those charged with developing population policy must be aware of the importance of the epidemic, and be able to incorporate the implications into their policy and projections.

■ There must be data on HIV prevalence in order for the potential size of the problem to be appreciated and for the epidemic to be modelled.

The South African Department of Welfare and Population Development has produced a White Paper on Population Policy.[18] The paper makes mention of HIV/AIDS, and indeed includes a special section: 2.3.4.4 HIV infection/AIDS. The section reflects on the size of the problem (although it uses out-of-date information), and the nature of the demographic and economic consequences. However, there is still no evidence that the consequences of the epidemic are being incorporated in projections, or that the consequences are being considered in a realistic and systematic manner.

Conclusion

The reason we are concerned about HIV and AIDS is that it causes people to fall ill and die. Measuring illness and its demographic impact is not easy; methods are being developed which look at issues such as the burden of disease and quality of life. These are complicated and need further refinement. Measuring the demographic impact of death is easier, but the broad picture depends on having regular population registration and censuses. At the moment, the latter are only held every 10 years. While demographers are supposed to take into account all factors in modelling future population trends, they have been slow to appreciate the consequences of AIDS for population forecasts. Of one thing they can be certain: there is about to be a significant rise in mortality in South Africa.

7 The economic, developmental and social impact of AIDS

An increase in illness and death in a population will inevitably have economic and social consequences. For each individual and his or her family, an HIV diagnosis and its consequences are a disaster. What is not clear is the degree to which AIDS will impact on the community and nation at the macro level. A hierarchy of organisation is shown in Chart 7.1.

Chart 7.1 Hierarchy of organisation

Social	Economic	Spatial
Individual	Consumer/producer	Living space
Family	Household	Home
Community	Unit of production	Village/neighbourhood
Tribe	Subsector	Town/city
Ethnic group	Sector	Province/region
Nation	National economy	Country
Mankind	Global economy	Earth

Note: This is indicative – there will be variations in countries and societies.

What will the impact of AIDS be in South Africa? Since the late 1980s, the doom-and-gloom merchants have been having a field day in predicting the dire consequences of the AIDS epidemic. This was epitomised in a book, *AIDS: Countdown to Doomsday*, published in 1988:[1] The author argued that AIDS was likely to lead to economic collapse and a shifting balance of global power. The reality is that the projections of global economic and social collapse have not and will not come true. In Africa, the epidemic is of a different order of magnitude and the impacts will be commensurately greater. But it is not entirely clear what they will be, as is apparent from the discussion in the rest of this chapter. In South Africa, the effect is only just beginning to be felt. There are a number of reasons for this:

■ South Africa is at the moment experiencing an HIV epidemic.

The AIDS epidemic is still developing. While the HIV epidemic is projected to peak around 2010 (it may even be sooner), AIDS cases will continue to grow for another 5 to 10 years. Chart 7.2 provides a timescale of the two epidemics.

■ Except at the micro or household level where the effect of AIDS is immediate, the economic impact will only slowly manifest itself as the number of individual illnesses and deaths accumulate over time. It may take even longer to show up in the official figures.

■ Ultimately, the economic impact will depend on how many people are infected and who they are. Economics does not value all lives equally. However, everyone is a consumer even if they are not producers.

■ Social impacts arise because people interact in ways other than economic. The complexity of this is illustrated in Chart 7.3.

Chart 7.2   A timescale for the epidemic

From – to (in years)	Minimum	Maximum
First AIDS case to peak of HIV in urban areas	12	25
Urban HIV peak to national HIV peak	8	10
National HIV peak to peak in AIDS cases	5	10
Impact on next generation	10	40
Total	**35**	**85**

MYTH

When HIV prevalence peaks, we can all relax because the main fury of the epidemic will be spent.

REALITY

HIV incidence may still be high when HIV prevalence peaks, but it is being offset by AIDS deaths. Moreover, the curve of AIDS cases can still be rising strongly and it is this one that really affects the economy.

Chart 7.3   The individual as an economic and social actor

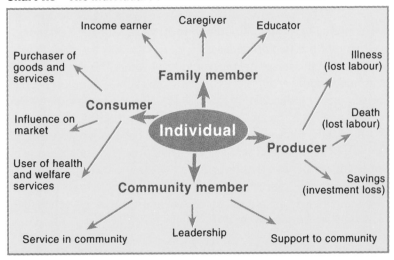

South Africa is at the beginning of the AIDS epidemic. The impact of illness and death is being felt by families, the public health service, and some private-sector firms. However, it will take time to work through into society at large. To find examples of impact, we have therefore to look to countries where the epidemic is further advanced. However, two caveats must be noted:

■ Even in the developing countries where the epidemic is most advanced, the impact is still evolving and is largely unknown.

■ South Africa is different to these countries. It is a more modern, skills-dependent and technologically advanced economy. Its citizens expect, and get, more from the state than is the case in most other African countries.

Despite these reservations, we can be sure of three things. The impact will be:

■ long-term
■ complex
■ surprising.

These points will be explored below.

MYTH

AIDS will solve the unemployment problem.

REALITY

By killing the economically active age group, AIDS will provide employment opportunities for those at present unemployed. Equally, AIDS will reduce the ranks of the unemployed as they fall sick and die. However, as will be seen later in this chapter, the effect of AIDS on economic growth is largely unknown at this stage. The impact on consumption may be so severe that the economy declines and people are put out of work as businesses downsize or close.

AIDS and national economic growth

Will AIDS have an impact on national growth? This is an important question as it is only through growth that redistribution can be funded and employment created. Furthermore, South Africa has experienced negative or very low growth for many years now. As South Africa is lagging behind other African countries in the epidemic, an obvious question is: what can be learnt from them? Unfortunately, surprisingly little. There have been attempts to model the macro-economic impact of AIDS, but they are fraught with difficulty. The models suggest that the mechanisms through which the epidemic may affect economies are:

■ The illness and death of productive people and the consequent fall in productivity.

■ The diversion of resources from savings (and eventually investment) to care. This will happen as people spend their savings on medication and special food and so on. As the disease progresses and financial resources are used up, people will begin cashing in insurance policies and selling capital items. In the rural areas, the sale of cattle and farming equipment is already known to occur.

The degree to which these factors will impact on national growth will depend on the people who are infected in terms of their importance to national production, and to what extent money is diverted from savings to care. It is a harsh *economic* reality that not all lives have equal value. If the majority of those who are infected are unemployed, subsistence farmers or unskilled workers, then the impact on the national economy will not be as great as if they are skilled and highly productive members of society. The same is true of savings. If the resources spent on care are considerable and come out of savings, then this will have a greater effect on the economy than if people do not spend money or the state provides the care. This complex issue was written about as early as 1992.[2] The paper showed that if the majority of people were unskilled and resources were not taken from savings to fund provision of care, then *in pure economic terms* the survivors could be better off and per capita income could rise! This conclusion is a political, moral and ethical hot potato, and discloses more about the limitations of pure economics than the impact of the epidemic.

MYTH
The epidemic will cause economic growth to falter and possibly even decline.
REALITY
This impact has not been seen anywhere. Models suggest that economic growth could slow as a result of AIDS, but this hypothesis still has to be proven.

There have been a number of models developed for the economic impact on specific countries, including Tanzania, Cameroon, and Zambia.[3] These models show that HIV may reduce the rate of economic growth and, over a period of 20 years, the reduction in GDP may be significant. For example, at the end of the period, the GDP may be up to 25 per cent lower than it would otherwise have been without AIDS. A recent report prepared by the Botswana Institute for Development Policy Analysis concluded that, over the next 10 years, Botswana's economy will be 31 per cent smaller than in an AIDS-free scenario.[4] However, in order to make these predictions, projections of both the AIDS epidemic and economic trends have to be combined. Both are difficult to model and combining them compounds the uncertainty. Moreover, it would appear that the dire macro-economic predictions associated with the onset of AIDS are contradicted by the continuation of high economic growth rates in Uganda (7,2 per cent per annum between 1990 and 1996 and 5,8 per cent in 1997/98), and Botswana (4,1 per cent per annum between 1990 and 1996 and 5,5 per cent for 1997/98).[5]

In South Africa, a study was done on the impact of AIDS on the national economy in 1991.[6] The study suggested that the major initial impact would be on the public health service. In the longer term, the epidemic was expected to pose a threat to ongoing economic growth, with some sectors being more seriously affected than others. The general conclusion was that while 'the overall effect of the AIDS epidemic would be a sustainable one for the South African economy for the next 15 years, the problem is still a *desperately serious* one for our society'.[7]

As South Africa enters the new century, it is clear that, in *macro-economic terms*, the epidemic is not yet having a measurable impact. However, the impact of AIDS is gradual, subtle and incremental. It may well be that we will only know the true impact on government and the private sector when we look back from 2010 at what actually happened. Even then, it will be necessary to isolate its effect from all the other factors that influence the economy, e.g. government economic policy, export markets, interest rates, etc.

Recently, South Africa was finally predicted to be at the threshold of renewed economic growth. In 2000 the economy was expected to grow by 3,5 per cent, and the growth rate was to remain over three per cent in the foreseeable future.[8] Will the increase in death and illness due to AIDS affect the prospects for economic growth in South Africa? The 2000 South African Budget Review produced by the Department of Finance includes a 'box' on population projections and HIV/AIDS. This notes that the effects of HIV/AIDS on future population growth and labour force participation are difficult to predict, as is the economic and social impact. However, it suggests that population growth may slow to close to zero per cent by 2010, with the growth of the working age population declining from over two per cent in 2000 to under 0,5 per cent by 2008.

The review paints a stark future in adding the following statement: 'The economic and social impact of HIV/AIDS is also hard to predict. Household structure and behaviour will change as the size, composition and productivity of the labour force are affected. HIV/

AIDS is more prevalent among the economically active part of the population, thus affecting economic activity through a loss of skills and experience. Labour productivity will decrease owing to absenteeism and illness of workers, and unit labour costs will increase as firms pay more for medical aid and group life or disability coverage. Initial evidence suggests that AIDS mainly affects lower income or skills groups (e.g. migrant or mobile labourers) but the future pattern is still unclear. One study predicts an HIV prevalence in 2003 of 12 per cent among highly skilled workers, 20 per cent among skilled workers and 27,2 per cent among low-skilled workers.

'Declining life expectancy and job losses in families will also affect the dependency ratio – the ratio of nonworking age population to the working population. More orphaned children and child-headed households, combined with fewer economically active people, will burden family support systems, with implications for the future development of South Africa's social security systems.'[9]

The Department of Finance is therefore beginning to take the threat of AIDS seriously. Over the next few years, we can expect a great deal more on this subject from them.

More recently ING Barings produced a report 'Economic Impact of AIDS in South Africa: A Dark Cloud on the Horizon'.[10] This combines earlier demographic modelling with macro-economic models. They noted that, although data were imperfect, the AIDS epidemic was expected to have an adverse impact on the South African economy. The 'nonalarmist' scenario suggested that annual GDP growth would be between 0,3 and 0,4 percentage points lower than the no-AIDS baseline over the next 15 years. The key areas identified by the report include:

■ South Africa is already battling with a skills shortage. AIDS will exacerbate this and raise remuneration and replacement costs for companies.

■ There will be a smaller labour force with lower productivity and income at the same time as demand grows for services such as health and welfare. Lower tax revenues combined with higher health spending will put pressure on the government's budget deficit. However, demand for housing as well as durable and non-durable goods could be negatively affected.

■ A rise in the inflation rate together with a smaller savings pool could well put pressure on interest rates.

■ Domestic savings may be squeezed to a point where foreign investment is vital to plug the gap. However, AIDS and the perception that it creates may deter such investment.

Meanwhile, the World Bank's paper 'Intensifying Action against HIV/AIDS: Responding to the Development Crisis' warns that a prevalence rate above five per cent not only makes the disease more expensive and difficult to contain; it also starts seriously reducing economic growth. We are double that threshold right now.[11]

Households

At the other end of the scale from the macro-economy is the household. Here, an AIDS case will always be traumatic and may be economically disastrous. The infected individual will require medical care and possibly special foods, thus increasing demands on household resources. At the same time, if the person is an adult, illness and death reduce household production capacity, resulting in a decline in household income. Thus, households are caught in a double bind of needing more resources at the very time when these may be reduced.

There are no studies in South Africa on the effect of AIDS on households. Indeed, there is surprisingly little information from other parts of the world either.[12] The most broadly based study of household responses to HIV/AIDS is the Kagera study from Tanzania. Unfortunately this has neither been fully analysed nor published.[13]

The overall economic impact of an adult death on surviving household members varies according to the characteristics of:

■ the deceased individual such as age, gender, income and cause of death;

■ the household itself, such as composition (number of adults and children and their ages) and assets (how much they have); and

■ the community such as attitudes towards helping needy households and the general availability of resources and standard of living in the community.[14]

One question which is often repeated is: will AIDS have a greater impact than death from other causes? The answer seems to be that it will – not least because of the stigma attached to this illness which can lead to individuals and households being excommunicated from society. Because of the protracted nature of HIV illness, there may be lengthy depletion of household resources giving rise to greater and more enduring hardship than other causes of death. A study by the Zimbabwe Farmers' Union in one communal and small farm area found that any adult death had an adverse affect on output; but, in the case of AIDS, it was worse. An adult death resulted in a 45 per cent decline in marketed output of maize. Where the cause of death was identified as AIDS, there was a 61 per cent loss. Marketed output of cotton declined by 20 per cent for an adult death and 47 per cent if the death was from AIDS.[15] There are similar findings on the impact of the disease from studies in Chiang Mai in Thailand, Abidjan in Côte d'Ivoire and various parts of Uganda.[16]

Most of these studies were intended, as the titles of their reports indicate, to be economic studies. However, they suffered from an inevitable problem: many of the seriously affected households had disappeared before the survey (and these were all survey-based studies) was undertaken.[17] This is likely to result in an under-estimation of the effects of epidemic illness and death because, in each case, the survey will be looking at households which have survived the earliest stages of the epidemic process. In addition, apart from the Thai and Côte d'Ivoire studies, no research has been commissioned on the impact of AIDS on households in urban areas, or more crucially and worryingly, in peri-urban areas and slums.

The South African population is, by African standards, highly urbanised with over 50 per cent of the population living in the urban areas. It is possible that the worst impacts may be in the urban and peri-urban areas. The reasons would be that there are no developed community support mechanisms; people are more impoverished; and they do not have access to food crops. Another possible problem area concerns the type of scheme whereby basic homes are provided to poor people in South Africa. The concept is that basic housing should be provided with the occupants paying towards the cost of their homes, and for utilities. If families are facing the loss of incomes and increased demands on their resources on account of AIDS, this may no longer be feasible. In addition, the design of homes may not be appropriate for a population facing an AIDS epidemic. The Provincial Housing and Development Board of KwaZulu-Natal issued a guideline, *AIDS: Provision of Housing*, on 2 November 1999. Noting that the Housing Act No. 107 of 1997 calls for all levels of government to 'promote the meeting of special housing needs, including, but not limited to, the needs of the disabled', and taking into account the extent of the HIV/AIDS crisis in KwaZulu-Natal, the Board said it would consider funding for the provision of accommodation for people and families affected by AIDS. This could take the form of cluster homes for orphans; transitional housing for destitute adults and children; and provision for home-based care.[18]

Poverty

The links between poverty and health are increasingly recognised and understood.[19] It is not clear that AIDS is simply a disease of poverty, although poverty undoubtedly helps drive the epidemic. In the early stages AIDS appears to infect the relatively well off: they have the disposable incomes that allow them to travel and, in the case of men, purchase sex. Of course more poor people are infected – because there are more poor – but it is likely that, as the epidemic evolves, they may be proportionately worse affected. What is clear is that AIDS increases poverty.

There has been one in-depth study of a rural village in Tanzania. This study shows that AIDS-affected households are generally pushed into poverty and the situation faced by many can only be described as desperate.[20]

In South Africa the poorest 40 per cent of households receive only 11 per cent of total income, while the richest 10 per cent receive 40 per cent. The poor (classified as the poorest 40 per cent of households) are defined as those earning less than R355 per adult per month. The ultra poor (the poorest 20 per cent of households) are those earning below R194 per adult per month. About 50 per cent of the population (21 million) live in the poorest 40 per cent of households and are therefore classified as poor. About 27 per cent of the population (11 million) live in the poorest 20 per cent of households and make up the ultra poor.[21] For these households an AIDS case will decrease income and increase the demands on existing sparse resources. In effect, AIDS has the potential to push households even deeper into poverty.

AIDS may also increase inequality. Part of the survival strategy will be to sell assets, but 'when richer households purchase assets from AIDS-stricken poorer households, the long-term impact may be to accentuate existing inequalities in the distribution of incomes and assets'.[22] The cost of the disease is also being shifted onto households in various ways:

■ Where workers who are too ill to work are retrenched or medically boarded, they lose most of their benefits. Ultimately, they have to rely on the state or their families.

■ State hospitals recognise that they are neither the appropriate location nor can they provide care for people with AIDS. These patients are discharged to be cared for at home which places an extra financial burden on the households.

■ People living in urban areas may return to their rural homes when they fall ill, but they can no longer access health services there.

AIDS and human development[23]

Measuring the macro-economic impact of AIDS is not possible because it has not yet been felt. Assessing the impact at the household level is problematic and there has been no research in South or indeed southern Africa. AIDS is predicted to increase poverty and inequality, but nobody has measured this. However, there is *one* place where the effect of the epidemic is beginning to be seen in official data, and this is the United Nations' measurement of human development.

The concept of 'human development' was introduced in 1990 in order to look beyond economic measures. The United Nations Development Programme states: 'The purpose of development is to create an enabling environment for people to enjoy long, healthy and creative lives'.[24] In order to measure the 'human development' for individual countries so that they could assess their own progress and compare themselves with each other, the Human Development Index (HDI) was developed. The HDI combines three basic indicators of human wellbeing: leading a long life; being knowledgeable and enjoying a decent standard of living. The idea is that these can be combined to give an index of human development. The HDI has already been touched on in Chapter 6 when we pointed out the effect that AIDS will have on the life-expectancy component of the index (see Chart 6.10).

Despite the fact that those working in the field recognised early on that AIDS was going to affect life expectancy, this realisation did not seem to reach mainstream demographers until recently. Up to the publication of the 1997 Human Development Report, the UNDP had not factored AIDS into its calculations. Even now, the HDI for a specific country is based on a *modelled* decrease in life expectancy rather than an *observed* decrease.

Models also predict that the disease will increase infant and child mortality rates, two other measures widely regarded as key development indicators (see Chart 6.9 for child mortality rates).

The unmeasured impact: the social consequences of the HIV/AIDS epidemic

If it is difficult to measure and assess the impact of AIDS on national economic growth, on households and on development, it is even harder to assess the social consequences. Much of what follows is speculative and the true effects will only become apparent as the epidemic unfolds. Three concepts are of value in understanding how the epidemic may have social consequences. These are civil society, social capital and socially reproductive labour.

Civil society

Civil society has already been defined as that part of society which occupies the space between the individual and the state; and the degree to which there is a perceived and acted-upon community of interest in a group or nation. It includes any grouping of people outside the household and workplace. The extent of civil society helps determine the functioning – economic, social and cultural – of the society.

Social capital

Social capital is essential for the existence of civil society. However, social capital feeds into more than civil society. This has been well explored by Robert Putnam in a classic study of Italy.[25] The definition of social capital here is 'features of social organization, such as trust, norms and networks, that can improve the efficiency of society by facilitating co-ordinated actions'. Social capital is productive as it makes it possible to achieve ends that would not otherwise be attainable by individuals alone. The classic South African example is the *stokvel*. In order for a *stokvel* to operate, members have to trust each other to remain in the association and make their contributions. This trust is the social capital of the *stokvel*. Social capital is in many respects the medium through which individuals operate collectively in order to thrive.

Socially reproductive labour

Socially reproductive labour refers to the work which goes into the production of social capital. One type of socially reproductive labour with which we are all familiar is the care and rearing of children. But there are many other types. On the one hand, the work of a woman in the informal sector is close to the type of economic activity which is measured by economists. On the other hand, the functions of a chief or sangoma may be difficult to conceive of in economic terms, yet they may have critical importance in growing social capital. Care of orphans is most certainly socially reproductive labour, not only in terms of their physical care but also in regard to their emotional and social development.

These are areas where losses are not easily measured by the instruments of economics or those of other social sciences. Premature loss of this kind of social capital or socially reproductive labour without its replacement is a major loss to society. At a time when so much attention is paid to the importance of civil society, loss of social reproductive labour adversely affects social capital, which in turn threatens the existence of civil society. But it goes beyond this. Many of us take for granted that children will normally be brought up in caring, nurturing environments. AIDS overturns this principle. The norm is no longer a two-parent family or, prominent in the African context, the extended family.

94

Children and orphans

Of particular concern, therefore, is the level of orphaning. South Africa's population is young: 54 per cent are below 25 years of age and 12 per cent are below five.[26] Changes in population structure where young to middle-aged adults are lost will result in large numbers of orphans, as well as children in adoptive families, growing up with less adult attention than might otherwise have been the case. In some situations, children will receive little or no adult attention. Such is the lot of increasing numbers of street children and the small but growing number of 'child-headed' households. Nearly one million South African children under the age of 15 will have lost their mothers to AIDS by 2005. This is estimated to increase to around two million by 2010, according to the Department of Health. The difficulties surrounding the definition of orphans were discussed in the previous chapter so that these figures, if anything, may underestimate the scale of the problem.

Studies have been conducted on the plight of orphans and their caretakers in various African countries. Among the findings are that: families which foster children in Kenya usually live below the poverty line; and orphan households in Tanzania have more children, are larger, and have less favourable dependency ratios. Children who lose a parent to AIDS suffer loss and grief like any other orphan. However, their loss is exacerbated by prejudice and social exclusion, and can lead to the loss of education and health care. Moreover, the psychological impact on a child who witnesses his or her parent dying of AIDS can be 'more intense than for children whose parents die from more sudden causes. HIV ultimately makes people ill but it runs an unpredictable course. There are typically months or years of stress, suffering or depression before a patient dies'.[27]

For a child living with a parent who has AIDS, the disease is especially cruel as HIV is sexually transmitted. Consequently, once one parent is infected, he or she is likely to pass it on to the other parent. Children who lose one parent to AIDS are thus at considerable risk of losing their remaining parent as well. For children, therefore, AIDS will, over time, cause a major diminution in social capital in the form of lack of social skills, knowledge and unclear expectations. It will also lead to detectable and quantifiable declines in levels of formal education.

A bleak future is predicted by Martin Schönteich of the Institute for Security Studies in Pretoria. He warns that 'AIDS and age will be significant contributors to an increase in the rate of crime in South Africa over the next ten to twenty years. There will be a boom in South Africa's orphan population during the next decade as the AIDS epidemic takes its toll. Growing up without parents, and badly supervised by relatives and welfare organisations, this growing pool of orphans will be at greater than average risk to engage in criminal activity. Moreover, in a decade's time every fourth South African will be aged between 15 and 24. It is within this age group where people's propensity to commit crime is at its highest.'[28]

Thus, an increasing number of AIDS orphans, who grow up without parental support and supervision, may turn to crime. 'Crime will increase because of the disintegration of the fabric of our society. It will be made worse by the lack of guidance, care and support for HIV-positive people, including children. Children orphaned by AIDS will have no role models in the future and they will resort to crime to survive.'[29]

A series of interviews undertaken in 1998 with young South African men serving jail sentences, or involved in crime, by the Centre for the Study of Violence and Reconciliation found that most of the interviewees were 'abandoned or kicked out of their homes, or . . . had to live with a stepfather or mother who rejected them. Many expressed feelings of being unloved.'[30] Schönteich argues that the major predictor of crime will be the age structure of the population. During the next ten to twenty years, the number of juveniles and young adults as a proportion of the general population will peak. This will exert an upward pressure on the crime rate as juveniles and young adults are proportionately more likely to commit crime than children or adults. At about the same time, South Africa will also experience a rapid increase in the number of children growing up with no parents or only one parent because of the effects of AIDS. Most will grow up without adequate parental supervision, guidance, and discipline under impoverished conditions – an environment which will increase their temptation to engage in criminal activity at an early age. In other parts of Africa, like Sierra Leone and Liberia, this neglect has already spawned a multitude of boy soldiers who are seen touting around rifles, rocket-launchers and other weapons.

Conclusion

While readers will find much of the material in this chapter depressing, it is not meant to create a state of resignation and helplessness. Although many of the impacts we have described are already in the pipeline, much will depend on the way we tackle the disease over the next few years. It is quite possible, if there is a proper call to arms for every individual and institution in our land to fight AIDS, that civil society will find strength in adversity. But that is the topic of the last chapter.

8 AIDS and the private sector

The private sector has a crucial role to play in achieving sufficient economic growth in South Africa to raise the general standard of living. It is the major source of employment, creates wealth, and supplies the population with food, clothing, housing and most essential (and nonessential) goods and services. As we have already observed, some private sector firms, particularly in KwaZulu-Natal and Gauteng, are beginning to feel the impact of AIDS. This is manifesting itself in increased illness and death in the workforce. Unfortunately there is little published information quantifying the impact on companies in South Africa. Indeed, throughout Africa there are only half a dozen such studies. It is possible that studies have been carried out by a number of companies for internal purposes, but we are unable to access these.[1]

How has AIDS affected and how will it affect the private sector, and what is this sector's role in responding to the epidemic? There are two realities facing managers:

■ There will be a steady increase in illness and death in South Africa and much of it among the working-age population.

■ There is little information on the impact AIDS does have on business, at least not in the public domain. Where there is information, it is hard to interpret.

MYTH

AIDS is a boon for the environment because there will be less people to mess it up.

REALITY

AIDS, by weakening the profitability of industry, will ensure that less money is around to fund conservation and antipollution programmes.

Evidence of impact

AIDS primarily kills young and middle-aged adults during their most productive years. This means that it is unlike any other disease with which companies have had experience. Unfortunately, there is little companies can learn from the experiences of others. There have been only a few attempts to quantify the effect of the disease on companies' productivity and profitability. Furthermore, the studies that have been done were for the most part carried out in the early to mid-1990s when HIV infection rates were climbing rapidly, but there was still relatively little AIDS-related morbidity or mortality. Secondly, each study defines or reports the costs of the epidemic in a different way, e.g. as a percentage of the wage bill or a percentage of profits. This makes comparison across companies and countries difficult. Finally, the published studies rely on national antenatal clinic prevalence data to estimate and project the prevalence in largely male workforces. Three reasons account for this approach: the taking and testing of blood of employees requires informed consent; the tests will not necessarily give a good sample; and they are complicated and expensive. The advent of saliva tests mean that such surveys can now be carried out, and indeed have been done by Eskom and by Debswana in Botswana – but the data have not been released.

MYTH

AIDS is a soft business issue best handled by the human resource function in the company.

REALITY

AIDS is going to have a significant impact on bottom-line profits and needs to be part and parcel of line management's strategic thinking and decision-making.

The effects of HIV/AIDS on business are reduced productivity, increased costs and loss of customers. Profits are being depressed by a number of factors:

■ Absenteeism is increasing not only because of the ill health experienced by employees, but also because workers take time off to care for their families (these demands are felt especially by women) and for funerals.

- The morale of the workforce is sagging.
- Sick workers are less productive at work and cannot carry out the more demanding physical jobs.
- Accidents occur more frequently because of fatigue in the workplace.
- Employees who die or retire on medical grounds have to be replaced; their replacements may be less skilled and experienced and therefore may require training.
- The average age and experience of workers fall as the proportion of new and younger recruits (novices in the mining industry) rises.
- Employers are increasing the size of their workforce to provide for deaths during apprenticeship and because of absenteeism generally.
- As skilled workers become scarcer, wages have to be increased for the limited pool available.
- The communities in the neighbourhood of a business are needing more support to weather the crisis.
- The costs of health care, medical aid, and hospitalisation are rising.
- Where companies have granted credit to. customers for purchases and those customers are dying of AIDS, the balance of the loans is having to be written off.
- Growth in the volume of sales, and in some cases the actual volume of sales itself, is declining as the market shrinks through sickness and death.

Absenteeism and deaths

The largest element of HIV and AIDS-related costs is absenteeism. A study of a bus company in Zimbabwe demonstrated that AIDS-related absenteeism accounted for 54 per cent of AIDS costs. This was followed by absenteeism due to HIV-related symptomatic illness at 35 per cent. Zambia's largest cement company reported that absenteeism for funerals increased 15-fold between 1992 and 1995. As a result, the company has restricted employee absenteeism for funerals to only those for a spouse, parent or child. Indeed, as long as five years ago, some Ugandan companies were reporting steep increases in absenteeism and turnover among workers. By the mid-1990s, the Uganda Railway Corporation had an annual employee turnover rate of 15 per cent, with more than 10 per cent of its workforce dead from AIDS-related illness.[2] Chart 8.1 shows that, in a study carried out across a number of countries, it was found that absenteeism accounted for 52 per cent of costs.

Chart 8.1   Distribution of increased labour costs due to HIV/AIDS by category[3]

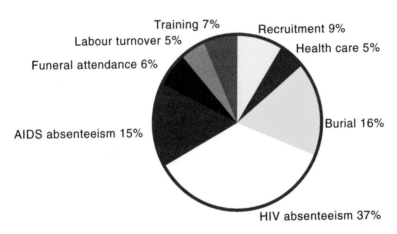

Ironically, even though mortality rates have risen, the direct costs of death are smaller than those for absenteeism: 16 per cent for burials and six per cent for funeral attendence. In Zambia, Barclays Bank has been losing 36 of its 1 600 employees each year, ten times the death rate of employees in companies in the West. In Kenya, out of the 50 employees of the Kenya Revenue Authority who died in 1998, 43 died from AIDS (i.e. 86 per cent). A 1996 study for the Makandi Tea Estate in Malawi showed a sixfold increase in mortality from 1991 to 1995 – from four per thousand workers to 23 per thousand.[4]

Employee benefits

In South Africa, a potentially significant area for additional AIDS costs relates to employee benefits. For individual companies, much will depend on the conditions of employment, the level of staff and what benefits are provided. Benefits typically include group life insurance, pensions, funeral benefits and medical aid. Essentially, there are two scenarios: either payroll costs will rise as is set out in the projection done by Metropolitan Life and shown in Chart 8.2; or benefits will be cut to contain costs.

Chart 8.2 Illustrative impact of AIDS on employee benefits in South Africa

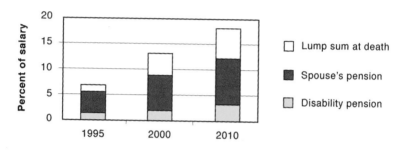

Case study: a sugar mill

One published case study in South Africa concerns the impact of HIV infection and AIDS deaths on a sugar mill with 400 workers, of whom 96 per cent are male.[5] It focused on how the disease affected workplace behaviour and calculated the consequential costs for the employer. The study was conducted at an occupational health clinic that oversees the primary care needs of the mill. The records of 23 workers who took ill-health retirement due to HIV during 1991-98 were inspected. The direct costs associated with HIV infection were estimated from records obtained from the occupational health clinic, hospital and insurance sources. Clinic visits, hospitalisations and treatments given were recorded for each patient. Ill-health and disability reports and records of employee attendance were also examined.

The study established monetary values for lost time due to illness, clinic visits and hospitalisation. The costs of HIV increased substantially in the last two years of employment, so the records were reviewed over this time period. The average number of days lost due to illness in the last two years prior to employees taking ill-health retirement was 55,5 days, or 27,7 days per year. A cost was applied for lost productivity, and for the recruitment and training of a new employee based on previous replacements. The total cost per worker per year for the period of the analysis was R9 543 with equal shares of 28 per cent for replacement worker costs, productivity losses and absenteeism (see Chart 8.3). The medical care and hospitalisation costs were minimal by comparison. This is very similar to the results for other African countries.

Chart 8.3 Direct cost of HIV/AIDS per worker per year

Cost:	Per cent of total
Replacement workers	28
Lost productivity	28
Training	5
Hospitalisation	1
Clinic and physician visits	10
Absenteeism	28
Total	**100**

The evidence suggests that the cost of the disease will depend on the type of company, the skill levels and replaceability of employees, the sector it operates in and the benefits it provides. The most seriously affected businesses might be those in labour-intensive industries, such as transportation, and those dependent on migrant workers such as mining. Certainly in Zimbabwe, which is further advanced in the epidemic, the main concerns of businesses were: the loss of skilled labour (33 per cent saw this as the key issue); the loss of labour generally (24 per cent); future reductions in productivity (24 per cent); increased insurance and pension costs (13 per cent); and other associated economic costs (12 per cent). Short-term concerns focused on the labour impacts of AIDS, including recruitment, training and development, and employee benefits; and long-term concerns focused on the way AIDS would affect the markets.

In South Africa, there has been one corporate survey (in 1998).[6] The researchers sent out questionnaires to 16 companies to get a clearer picture of their response to AIDS. The questionnaire asked what impact HIV/AIDS had had on the company; whether they had had to deal with any HIV/AIDS-related problems/issues; and whether they knew of any HIV-positive people in the company. Only four companies responded! Impala Platinum mine estimated that 17 per cent of workers were HIV positive and an average of four employees per month were dying. The Natal-based Tongaat-Hulett Group reported that 17 per cent of all ill-health retirements in 1997 had AIDS as the diagnosis, and there was a 31 per cent increase in ill-health retirements from 1995. Woolworths and Naspers reported no impact. Until recently, the vast majority of companies were not considering HIV/AIDS as an important business issue. Restructuring, economic uncertainty and new labour legislation were the overriding concerns. Anglo American, however, has recently published a report on its response to the AIDS crisis in southern Africa.[7] It includes Chart 8.4, which analyses the requirements of a comprehensive HIV-prevention programme. Progress against this programme is being regularly assessed throughout the Group's operations.

Chart 8.4   Key elements essential to a comprehensive HIV-prevention programme

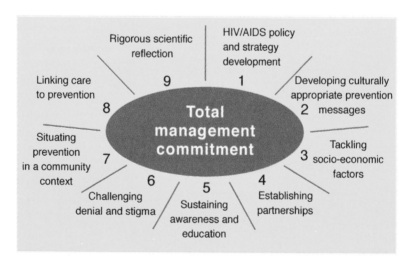

Impact on markets

HIV/AIDS could reduce the absolute number of potential customers, making markets that are relatively saturated and which depend critically on population growth the most vulnerable. While in some countries total population growth over the next decade might remain positive, growth will be markedly slower. The impact of the epidemic on specific markets will depend on the demographic profile (e.g. age, sex, income level, geographic location) of consumers. Where demand for goods is far from saturated and growing strongly, many of the consumers who die or have their disposable income reduced by HIV/AIDS will be replaced by new earners and consumers. Yet even the strongest markets will wilt if overall GDP and consumption expenditure are badly hit by the epidemic.

In South Africa, labour market adjustments to HIV/AIDS, such as increasing capital intensity or using less skilled labour that is cheaper to replace, may exacerbate economic and political polarisation. Market growth for goods and services targeted at upwardly mobile households may also be severely affected. A major concern for the retail sector in South (and southern) Africa is the provision of credit. Many of the clothing chains offer credit which is written off in the event of the customer's death. In addition, store cardholders may be offered funeral benefits in the event of their or their dependants' deaths. An article in *AIDS Analysis Africa* reported that 'an insurance company in Durban, which underwrites claims on death and funeral benefits of a major retail chain, reported a 50 per cent increase in the number of claims last year (1998). Steps are being taken to increase premiums in line with the expected increase in deaths.'[8] Retailers of household appliances and furniture will also be affected since many of these goods are sold on hire purchase. Although customers are required to buy life insurance, there is likely to be a higher frequency of defaults.

It must, however, be recognised that, for some businesses, AIDS represents an opportunity. These include the providers of health care, the burial industry and AIDS NGOs and activists.

Case study: the JD Group

One company that has looked at the potential impact of the epidemic on their markets and customer base, and considered how to reposition itself in the light of this, is the JD Group (JDG). They were prepared to share their findings at a recent conference on AIDS in Cape Town. JDG sells furniture and household appliances. Stores include Bradlows, Russells, Electric Express and Score as well as Joshua Doore.[9]

The study was done in 1998 and looked at issues around the development of a new product range; marketing strategies; the opening and relocation of stores; lease negotiations for stores; and employee profiles and benefits. The report looked at the epidemic from a business point of view and included a forecast of HIV prevalence among customers by market segment and store group. It is believed that the overall HIV prevalence rate among JDG's customers is currently 15 per cent and this will rise to 27 per cent by 2015. The data are shown in Chart 8.5, and match most predictions of the likely trends in the epidemic.

Chart 8.5   HIV prevalence rate in JD Group customers

Year	2000	2005	2010	2015
Prevalence rate (%)	15	23	26	27

The report concluded that the South African customer base would grow slowly until 2010. Thereafter, the demographic impact of AIDS would kick in, resulting in an 18 per cent decline in customers by 2015 in all provinces bar the Western Cape. Other countries such as Swaziland, Lesotho and Botswana would experience a reduction in market size by 2010 of about 14 per cent.

The increase in illness and death means that consumption patterns will change as disposable income is reallocated. Such an action will thereafter have a knock-on effect on the granting of credit because customers' creditworthiness may well be impaired. As JDG makes its money on credit sales as well as cash sales, a potential increase in defaulting by borrowers is cause for concern. In the longer term, industry-specific worries may be aggravated by a rise in interest rates and inflation. The latter would be brought on by additional spending on AIDS care in both the public and private sectors. Government itself could be forced to spend less on housing and infrastructure.

All this spells bad news for the local retail sector. JDG concluded that:

■ The epidemic will influence consumption patterns as households divert expenditure to AIDS care.

■ The previous relationships between GDP, personal consumption expenditure and durable consumption expenditure will change.

■ Considerable social impact is expected of the kind we explained in the previous chapter.

■ The impacts by age group and market region are anticipated to differ substantially.

■ A strategic repositioning of the JD Group will be required before 2005.

The study was done so that the company could incorporate the HIV scenario into its strategic thinking. JDG took various decisions including that of remaining within its core competencies and strengthening its market position[10]; that of leveraging its existing infrastructure to cater for other customer needs; and that of diversifying geographically away from the HIV/AIDS epidemic. As a result, it has introduced personal services as part of the product range it offers and has expanded into Eastern Europe. Jan Bezuidenhout, an Executive Director of JDG, is emphatic that the company remains committed to South Africa. Equally, however, it has a responsibility to its shareholders to safeguard its future income stream. The opening of stores in Poland and the Czech Republic ensures that the future income sources will be diversified and JDG's return to shareholders will remain reasonable.

JDG is the only major retailer to have carried out a study of the impact of AIDS. As Mr Bezuidenhout noted, this has led to some competitors ridiculing them. Nevertheless, JDG's management have built the company by having the courage and vision to look ahead. They see AIDS as a sufficient problem to take seriously and plan for it. If the epidemic turns out to be not as bad as they fear, then no harm will have been done. If it fulfils predictions, they will survive.

The business environment

It is likely that AIDS will also have indirect impacts on the business community. Examples of this are:

■ The private sector may be able to adapt to absenteeism and the death of employees. However governments are less able to do so; and the result may be increasing government inefficiency, which leads to delays in granting licences, approving applications and so on.

■ Service providers may operate less efficiently; it is reported from Zambia that the increase in mortality among employees of its electricity corporation has resulted in interruptions to the electricity supply.

■ Trade unions may mobilise and make demands around HIV issues (although co-operation with the unions in an area like this can also be beneficial to the employer).

■ The increase in orphans and street children may increase the rate of crime which will make it more difficult to retain skilled but internationally mobile staff.

■ The police and defence force may experience increased mortality, particularly at the middle levels, which could decrease stability.

■ The state health system will experience much higher demands being placed on it, which may lead to a deterioration in the level and quality of service. This could put pressure on the private sector to use private hospitals to care for employees.

■ Government resources may be diverted from infrastructural projects, crucial to the functioning of the private sector, into care and prevention programmes.

■ A concern peculiar to South Africa is the impact on affirmative action. For historical reasons, the levels of infection are higher in the black population than the white. The national policy of affirmative action is likely to be hindered by the AIDS mortality.

■ In other African countries, there are likely to be problems around localisation policies. Many countries have spent years developing local skills to replace expatriates. AIDS may delay and reverse the implementation of these programmes. A more worrying problem is that government policies may not recognise the new realities.

It should be noted that the last two points have been largely ignored as they are politically problematic. But they need to be addressed.

Models for assessing costs to business

What can and should companies do about AIDS? The first step is to look at what AIDS will mean to the company. While there may be a shortage of case studies to learn from, one has to start by making a careful quantitative assessment of the additional costs incurred in maintaining a productive workforce. There are a number of examples of how the impact of the epidemic might be assessed.

While these assessments are not conceptually complicated, they do require a large amount of data. The latter can only be obtained from the companies themselves, and with a significant investment in the analysis. In this section, we look at models to identify the additional costs which businesses will have to bear.[11]

The first, depicted in Chart 8.6, is a chronological model designed to alert business managers to all the steps required to cope with the spread of HIV/AIDS among employees, and to assist them in capturing all the financial implications associated with the disease. The bottom line is that HIV/AIDS will make it more expensive for a company to produce a given quantity of its product unless it can reduce its costs in other ways. If there is no fat to be cut, the company will either have to raise prices, market its product more aggressively or accept a reduction in profits. Should the increase in HIV/AIDS-related costs be large enough, the company may face the prospect of going out of business, causing all of its employees to lose their jobs and incomes. Obviously, top management will seek to avert such a catastrophe by formulating a new strategic plan (like the JD Group did).

For purposes of data collection and analysis, the costs identified in Chart 8.6 can be reconfigured into a second model, depicted in Chart 8.7. This includes three types of costs. 'Direct costs' refer to impacts that involve increased financial outlays by the company. 'Indirect costs' reflect reduced workforce productivity (less output for a given level of expenditure on labour). These include reduced productivity by both the infected employee and by other employees who are diverted from their normal responsibilities. And finally,

109

Chart 8.6 Progression of cases and costs of workforce HIV/AIDS

Progression of HIV/AIDS in the workforce	Economic impact of individual case	Economic impact of all cases
1 Employee becomes infected with HIV virus	■ No costs to company at this stage	■ No costs to company at this stage
2 HIV/AIDS-related morbidity begins	■ Sick leave and other absenteeism increase ■ Work performance declines due to employee illness ■ Overtime and contractors' wages increase to compensate for absenteeism ■ Use of company's on-site health clinics increases ■ Payouts from medical aid schemes increase ■ Employee requires attention of human resource and employee assistance personnel	■ Overall productivity of workforce declines ■ Overall labour costs increase ■ Additional use of medical aid benefits causes premiums to increase ■ Additional medical staff must be hired at the company's health clinics ■ Managers begin to spend time and resources on HIV-related issues ■ HIV/AIDS interventions are designed and implemented
3 Employee leaves workforce due to death, medical boarding, or voluntary resignation	■ Payout from death benefit or life insurance scheme is claimed ■ Pension benefits are claimed by employee or dependants ■ Other employees are absent to attend funeral ■ Funeral expenses are incurred ■ Company loans to employee are not repaid ■ Co-workers are demoralised by loss of colleague	■ Payouts from pension fund cause employer and/or employee contributions to increase ■ Returns on investment in training are reduced ■ Morale, discipline, and concentration of other employees are disrupted by frequent deaths of colleagues

'systemic costs' refer to costs that result from the cumulative impact of multiple HIV/AIDS cases.

Most direct costs can be readily measured using human resources

Progression of HIV/AIDS in the workforce	Economic impact of individual case	Economic impact of all cases
4 Company recruits a replacement employee	■ Company incurs costs of recruitment ■ Position is vacant until new employee is hired ■ Cost of overtime wages increases to compensate for vacant positions	■ Additional recruiting staff and resources must be brought in ■ Wages for skilled (and possibly unskilled) employees increase as labour markets respond to the loss of workers
5 Company trains the new employee	■ Company incurs costs of pre-employment training (tuition, etc.) ■ Company incurs costs of in-service training to bring new employee up to level of old one ■ Salary is paid to employee during training	■ Additional training staff and resources must be brought in
6 New employee joins the workforce	■ Performance is low while new employee comes up to speed ■ Other employees spend time providing on-the-job training	■ There is an overall reduction in the experience, skill, institutional memory and performance of the workforce ■ Work unit productivity is disrupted as labour turnover rates increase

and financial data that large companies routinely collect. Indirect costs are much more difficult to measure. Some, such as the costs of absenteeism and morbidity, are measurable in theory; the difficulty lies in generating relevant data. For on-the-job morbidity, for example, estimates are needed of the percentage loss of productivity experienced by the sick worker and the duration of the productivity loss. Estimating the opportunity cost of management time devoted to HIV/AIDS-related issues is even more difficult.

Systemic costs are the most difficult to measure, especially in the short run and for individual companies. They include the toll that

Chart 8.7   Economic impact on workforce of HIV/AIDS

Direct costs

Benefits package
- Company-run health clinics
- Medical aid/health insurance
- Disability insurance
- Pension fund
- Death benefit/life insurance payout
- Funeral expenses
- Subsidised loans

Recruitment
- Recruiting expenses (advertising, interviewing, etc.)
- Cost of having positions vacant (profit the employee would have produced)

Training
- Pre-employment education and training costs
- In-service and on-the-job training costs
- Salary while new employee comes up to speed

HIV/AIDS programmes
- Direct costs of prevention programmes (materials, staff, etc.)
- Time employees spend in prevention programmes
- Studies, surveys, and other planning activities

Indirect costs

Absenteeism
- Sick leave
- Other leave taken by sick employees
- Bereavement and funeral leave
- Leave to care for dependants with AIDS

Morbidity on the job
- Reduced performance due to HIV/AIDS sickness on the job

Management resources
- Managers' time and effort for responding to workforce impacts, planning prevention and care programmes, etc.
- Legal and human resource staff time for HIV-related policy development and problem solving

Systemic costs

Loss of workplace cohesion
- Reduction in morale, motivation, and concentration
- Disruption of schedules and work teams or units
- Breakdown of workforce discipline (slacking, unauthorised absences, theft, etc.)

Workforce performance and experience
- Reduction in average level of skill, performance, institutional memory, and experience of workforce

Direct costs ➡ | Indirect costs ⬇ Total costs of HIV/AIDS in the workforce ⬅ | Systemic costs

illness and death among co-workers take on employee morale and motivation; the increases in occurrences of slacking and theft; and the overall loss of experience and skills in the workforce. The practical impossibility of measuring these costs in most cases should not be taken as a sign that they are not significant or can be omitted

112

from a company's strategy in coping with the epidemic. On the contrary, these costs could in the long run pose the most serious threat to companies' profitability.

Estimating aggregate costs in all three categories (as opposed to the costs of an individual infection) requires three other critical pieces of information. First, HIV/AIDS prevalence, morbidity, and mortality must be either measured (through voluntary, anonymous testing) or modelled. Second, because HIV infection rates tend to vary with age, sex, race, geographic location within South Africa and by job level, a detailed demographic profile of the current and future workforce is critical to the analysis. Finally, certain positions and skills are vital to a company's core processes. If such positions are vacant, the ability to provide the product or service will be heavily or completely impaired. These critical positions and skills have to be identified upfront and the people filling them carefully monitored for illness.

Once all the potential influences that HIV/AIDS could have on a company's internal and external environment have been ascertained, suitable responses to the challenge have to be formulated. These fall into four areas:

The impact on production and employees. In order to ensure that the production process is not vulnerable to staff losses, responses might include multiskilling, recruiting and training additional labour, contracting out, and capital intensification. In addition, the company should seek to prevent its workers from becoming infected through education and training, through provision of condoms and health services, and through examining the root causes of HIV transmission and addressing them. There are many examples of education and condom programmes which show that a reduction in levels of STDs will bring HIV infections down. Companies, therefore, need to recognise that their employees are members of the community. This is where transmission occurs and where interventions should primarily take place. Some tough questions have to be asked about the root causes of transmission. For example, does a company employ single male migrants, or are the employees required to spend large amounts of time away from their families? It may be possible to replace migrants with local people or reduce the time workers spend away from home. This requires imagination and lateral thinking.

The impact on costs. The costs of the disease need to be monitored and either reduced or accepted. It should be remembered that although a company may be able to reduce its costs by, for example, cutting back on medical benefits, these costs will have to be borne by someone somewhere. The state may be forced to step in or communities and households, already under pressure, will have to provide care.

The impact on markets. The effect of increased illness on markets is a major issue for companies which sell most of their products and services locally. Exporters to markets overseas may not have a similar problem. At the very least, a company should do what the JD Group did and assess the composition of its customers, their vulnerability to contracting the disease and how they will react in terms of changing their expenditure patterns.

Business in society. AIDS is such a serious and far-reaching problem that it will define how societies develop over the first half of the new century in Africa. Business cannot distance itself from the society in which it operates. In fact, the degree to which a company is socially responsible is now a critical element in the evaluation of that company by the public. There has been a lot of emphasis in recent years about forming partnerships against AIDS. The idea is that there should be a coalition against the epidemic involving government, business, trade unions, NGOs and the broader civil society. But what does it mean and how can it be moved forward in the African setting?

We all know (and have come to accept) that the business of business is business. It is not the job of business to run country-wide awareness campaigns, though they may be requested to participate in the funding. If the private sector is to be involved in a partnership, it must be made very clear as to what the role of each stakeholder is. Moreover, each role should play to that stakeholder's strength. People are less effective if called upon to do things lying outside their normal field of competency. Nevertheless, for a partnership to work, there has to be give and take on all sides.

For example, if tax breaks are provided for training (as is the case in most countries), should they not be provided for AIDS awareness programmes? How can government and business share best practice among themselves in terms of prevention and treatment programmes? How can drug companies assist the government in making current therapies universal and affordable? Can the government exempt all AIDS therapies from VAT and import duties in exchange? How can the advertising industry help in creating a campaign that connects with the learners in primary and secondary schools? The starting point would be to identify the key elements of an anti-AIDS programme and see who is most competent to do what.

At a very minimum, there should be a company policy on HIV/AIDS covering prevention, care and nondiscrimination. It should include practical management strategies, workplace principles and a workplace programme which has universal buy-in from employees. Ideally, the company will have a mission statement on AIDS and include the community in its response.

Interventions can work: the Lesedi project[12]

The Lesedi project began in Virginia in 1996. This Free State town is home to 80 000 people of whom 13 000 are miners, most living in single-sex hostels and working at the Harmony mine. The project involved Harmony Gold Mining Company and the provincial and national departments of health and was supported by USAID and Pfizer Pharmaceuticals. Additional support came from the South African National Reference Centre for STDs and the Antwerp Institute of Tropical Medicine.

The intervention comprised treatment of STDs in miners; monthly treatment of women at high risk of infection; sexual health promotion; counselling; and promotion of male and female condom use. The results have been impressive. The prevalence of genital ulcers among miners fell from 5,7 per cent to 1,3 per cent. Among women the decrease was from 10 per cent to 3,3 per cent. Gonorrhoea prevalence fell from 14,6 per cent to eight per cent among women and chlamydia from 13,5 per cent to 2,9 per cent. It was estimated that by 1999 an estimated 235 HIV infections had been averted (a 46 per cent decrease). These would have cost R2,34 million, whereas the cost of the intervention was R268 000!

The message is that averting HIV infection through prevention programmes can be very cost-effective.

MYTH
AIDS prevention and treatment programmes are very costly.
REALITY
The cost of doing nothing will shortly outweigh the cost of intervention.

The treatment issue

With the cost of medical treatments coming down, one major issue is rearing its head. It is quite possible that the cost of *nontreatment* of employees will soon be higher than the cost of *treatment*. However, for a treatment programme to be properly implemented, the question is: how can, and should, one undertake tests of the whole workforce to establish which individuals are HIV positive and which are not? If this were done, therapies could be introduced sooner rather than later for those who tested positive and, if needs be, they could be moved to less physically demanding occupations where their health was less at risk. Those who tested negative could be given intense education courses on ways to prevent themselves from becoming infected. Such a course of action, particularly if it is done in full consultation with employees, is quite different to pre-employment testing, against which a case of discrimination may be mounted justifiably.

However, two issues remain:

■ Would the private sector provide different levels of care depending on the value of the employee to the company?
■ If the private sector is prepared to look after all its employees with the latest therapies, what about the other people in South Africa who do not have access to them?

There are no easy solutions. However, these issues have to be addressed and, given the rapid development in treatment regimes, the sooner the better.

The law and HIV/AIDS

Law governing the manner in which employers handle HIV and AIDS matters in the workplace is still in its infancy. The Employment Equity Act is the only Act which expressly refers to HIV and AIDS. It prohibits unfair discrimination against the employee on the grounds of HIV status. It also bars medical testing except under special circumstances, and then, on one interpretation, only with the authorisation of the Labour Court. It is not yet clear exactly what those circumstances are or what role the Labour Court will play in giving or withholding its permission for testing. There are plenty of other laws in fields such as labour, health and safety which will impinge on companies and where they will have to check for compliance. Appendix 2 gives a more detailed picture of the unfolding legal situation.

9 AIDS and nation building

It is ten years since F.W. de Klerk made his historic speech un-banning the ANC and the SACP; releasing Nelson Mandela; and setting South Africa on the road to multiparty democracy. Despite many trials and tribulations, the first open elections were held in 1994 and it appears that democracy and government through the ballot box are firmly entrenched in South Africa. The government's economic policies are beginning to bear fruit and reasonable economic growth is forecast for the next three years.

One of the key issues for the new government was to begin the task of nation building. This was, in part, achieved through the Truth and Reconciliation Commission (TRC). The hearings brought home to many just how abhorrent the activities of the apartheid regime had been (although the liberation movements also had actions to answer for). Like a Greek tragedy used to have a cathartic effect on its audience, so the litany of horrors revealed by the TRC was part of the healing process for us. 'Never again' is not a bad message with which to start building a new nation. Yet fate has dealt South Africa a cruel blow by replacing apartheid with HIV as public enemy number one.

Since 1994, the government has moved rapidly to expand services such as health and education. Indeed, health care was made free for pregnant women and children under the age of six, and education enshrined as a constitutional right. Provision of potable water, electricity and housing were national priorities and, under the Reconstruction and Development Programme, ambitious targets were set. Of course all this had to be paid for, and not through increasing government borrowing or raising taxes. It was always intended that, with the exception of the health care mentioned above, the beneficiaries should pay at least part of the costs. HIV has made it inordinately difficult for poor people to fork up their share.

In 1994, South Africa was a divided country. Apart from the

118

obvious racial tensions there were deep political divisions as well. At the extreme, in places like KwaZulu-Natal, these divisions have at times surfaced in bitter and bloody conflict between the rival parties. HIV and AIDS love sporadic wars like this because they emerge as the only victor. Messages about a long-term threat like AIDS have no validity in situations where homes are being burned and people terrorised.

Meanwhile, in the urban areas, part of the struggle tactic was to make the townships ungovernable. The stratagem worked. However, re-establishing the rule of law has not been easy. The widespread availability of weapons, lack of legitimacy of the police (even now) and high unemployment rate among the youth have made it harder still. The absence of civil society and individual responsibility creates an environment conducive to the spread of HIV and one in which prevention messages become difficult to convey and act on.

All in all, HIV could not have had more welcoming surroundings in which to make its debut in South Africa. At last, we are responding, but the perception of many is that the response has been inadequate, flawed and inappropriate. How does this bear up to examination?

The government response

The first meaningful response to AIDS emerged with the birth of the National AIDS Convention of South Africa (NACOSA). In October 1992, a national conference entitled 'South Africa United Against AIDS' was addressed by Nelson Mandela. The purpose of the event was to launch the development of a national AIDS strategy to be followed by an implementation plan. Every significant sector was involved and NACOSA set about its task. The scale of the job, the pace at which it was done and the ability of adversaries from the apartheid days to work together set it apart as a unique achievement.

In October 1994, Minister Nkosazana Zuma, as Minister of Health in the new democratic government, accepted the NACOSA plan as the blueprint for the Government's AIDS Programme. However, there were major flaws in the NACOSA plan – not in the contents, which are still valid today, but in the lack of attention to

119

process and the failure to acknowledge the realities of the social, political and economic situation in South Africa at the time. In effect, there was no 'reality check', a fundamental principle of good planning. For example, the NACOSA budget was R257 million, more than ten times the 1994 national AIDS budget. Even if the funds had been available, the human resources were not and it would never have been possible to meet the targets in the Plan. Generally, though, the country was entering a period of transformation where AIDS would need to compete for attention with other critical issues. The net result was a suboptimal response:

■ confounded by the constant restructuring of the units at national and provincial level responsible for leading the response;
■ impeded by the devolution of the task of implementation from the national level to the provinces where capacity was extremely limited; and
■ complicated by 'AIDS politics'.

Each of these three factors bears examining.

Restructuring

Prior to 1995, the main public sector structures with responsibilities for AIDS were an AIDS Unit in the National Department of Health and about 12 AIDS Training, Information and Counselling Centres or ATICCs, located in the larger cities. The AIDS Unit generated masses of small media materials; some were quite effective, but some were very problematic such as posters with completely different messages for different population groups. The ATICCs, funded by the AIDS Unit, evolved along different lines in different parts of the country, but all had the core functions described in their name. They developed additional functions in accordance with the expertise of their staff: media development, research, outreach projects and so on. This became their strength, particularly where communication and collaboration between the ATICCs was good. However, it should be noted that, at this stage, the response and responsibility were firmly located in the health sector.

120

Devolution

The issue of devolution proved to be a significant barrier to progress and expansion, particularly in the public sector. That it needed to happen was never in dispute; the powers of provinces and the assignment of functions are constitutionally defined. However, what it meant in effect was that an extra layer of officials came into being at provincial level, many of whom were new to the field of AIDS and remained in their new positions for months, if not years, in an acting capacity. In early 2000, of those who took up these positions, only two of the original provincial co-ordinators were still in place.

In addition, funds for AIDS could no longer be 'ring-fenced' and directed from national government to the provinces and then to magisterial districts to be spent on specific projects. Budgetary decisions were taken in each province without any real reference to national priorities. Provinces received a global budget for all their functions and this had to be divided up between the different departments. As at national level, AIDS fell under the Provincial Health Departments and competed with other health priorities for funds and staff. This resulted in AIDS having very different profiles in different provinces. Furthermore, AIDS was still perceived as a health sector issue.

Politics

Then we have the matter of 'AIDS politics'. It has always been a part of South Africa's AIDS history. In 1995, the Sarafina II scandal erupted. The idea was to build on the success of the film *Sarafina* (which starred Whoopi Goldberg) and produce a musical stage production with an AIDS message which would tour the country. Whilst the motivation for the play might have been sound – to mobilise the youth who had been so effective during the struggle – it was, ultimately, nothing more than a lavish production of questionable value in terms of AIDS awareness. Moreover, irregularities were proven in the awarding of the tender. All in all, the debacle caused major dismay and alienation in the NGO sector which up to that time had been supportive of the Minister and the Department of Health.

121

Barely a year later, Virodene, the wonder treatment that came to be nothing hit the front pages and was, instantly, and even in the remotest corners of the country, the most sought-after 'remedy'. The researchers were initially supported at the highest political level, and only after extensive processes by the Medicines Control Council was the testing of Virodene on humans finally outlawed. Virodene contained dimethyformamide (DMF), an industrial solvent which was meant to block HIV. But it is also a toxic chemical known to cause liver damage in humans.

The furore over Virodene only dissipated when another matter emerged to take its place. There was to be compulsory, but anonymous, notification of everyone diagnosed with AIDS (not HIV) to the Department of Health. Furthermore, named notification would be provided to the immediate family, caregivers and anyone dealing with the person. Despite announcements in Cabinet and notices in the Government Gazette, this has not to date been implemented.

The 1997 review and more recent events

In mid-1997, a national review of South Africa's response to the AIDS epidemic was published entitled: *Review the Past, Plan the Future, Work Together*. The review findings highlighted the need for:
■ political leadership and public commitment;
■ meaningful involvement of people living with HIV and AIDS in policy formulation;
■ responses to be interdepartmental and intersectoral;
■ widespread capacity building;
■ close collaboration with the TB Programme; and
■ an urgent address of human rights abuses and the reduction of stigmatisation.

In the period immediately following the review, there was a unity of direction and purpose not experienced since the early NACOSA days. This momentum, however, was rapidly lost as the aforementioned Virodene and compulsory notification controversies divided constituencies and absorbed energies. But, in 1998, the political leadership and commitment so earnestly sought took the form of the Government AIDS Action Plan. A new staffing structure was established in the national Department of Health; the Interministerial Committee on AIDS was formed and a major public awareness campaign took place.

The main event that year was the address to the nation by President Mbeki on 9 October. In it, he confronted South Africans with the reality of the epidemic and called for sectors to pledge themselves to the Partnership Against AIDS. Various sectors (business and labour, youth and women, churches and faith communities, sport and entertainment) immediately stepped forward to articulate their commitment. But their enthusiasm faltered as they sought to identify their roles and to access capacity and financial assistance for implementation. Since then, events such as World AIDS Day, National Women's Day and Condom Week have become focal points for a wide range of awareness activities.

The one controversy which has carried across from Minister Zuma's to Minister Tshabalala-Msimang's administration has been the government's reluctance to approve access to short-course antiretroviral treatments for infected pregnant women. It is to be hoped that this matter can be satisfactorily resolved in the near future. Nevertheless, the country continues to be divided by misunderstandings and disputes. These have arisen from ill-advised pronouncements on the toxicity of antiretroviral drugs; a suggestion that treatment of pregnant women is uneconomic because they will leave orphans; and most worrying, the reopening of as basic an issue as whether HIV is the cause of AIDS. The last development will inevitably divert energy and money away from the real priority for South Africa, which is implementing a swathe of action programmes aimed at prevention and care. We don't have the luxury of time for too much contemplation on the origin of AIDS. As this edition goes to print, it has been reported that a small research subcommittee has been appointed by the government's international panel of experts to which reference is made later in this chapter. The objective of this subcommittee, which is made up of both mainstream and dissident scientists, is to devise a series of experiments which will settle the controversy once and for all.[1] Let us hope they do so!

The question is: why have we been so erratic in our responses to the AIDS epidemic? The answers are complex and we can only hypothesise about some of the reasons. Perhaps the single most important reason is that HIV was invisible for so many years. It could therefore be ignored by those who did not understand the implications of the rising prevalence rates. Linked to this was the perception that it was a *health* issue; as such, health personnel in both the public and private sectors were seen as having the responsibility of dealing with it. Unfortunately, health officials have neither the overall perspective, span of control nor the resources to deal with HIV. In most other African countries, it is recognised that HIV prevention and AIDS impact mitigation require a *multisectoral* response, although in fairness the realisation is neither automatic nor easy. Other issues that complicate responses by the nation are:

■ There is no single, simple answer to the epidemic – no magic bullet.

■ There are no all-embracing technical solutions.

■ The response will be long-term, and success will be hard to measure.

■ It is not clear how responses should be developed.

■ AIDS is bad news and dealing with it means addressing many of the issues around male sexuality and power – not something South African males (of all races) are comfortable with.

■ AIDS is jostling for priority with many other – apparently more important – development issues.

Success stories

The barriers, constraints and controversies are only one side of the picture. Many notable achievements bear mentioning.

Late in 1995, led by the newly restructured AIDS Directorate in the Department of Health, a renewed effort was made to identify key priorities. Five strategies were identified which, in time, were widely embraced by Government and many NGOs. These were:

■ Life-skills programmes targeted at the youth;

■ the use of mass communication to popularise key prevention concepts;

■ appropriate treatment and management of clients seeking treatment for STDs;

124

- increased access to barrier methods such as condoms; and
- the promotion of appropriate care and support.

Extensive funding was made available from both government and outside donors, primarily the European Union; and AIDS was given the status of a Presidential Lead Project which resulted in substantial additional funding from the Reconstruction and Development Programme. Unfortunately, this sudden injection of funds to government coincided with the withdrawal of donor funds to NGOs. In consequence, this period saw the demise of many AIDS Service Organisations, notably the AIDS Programme of the National Progressive Primary Health Care Network. Other NGOs, however, survived, including Soul City and Puppets Against AIDS, which have made valuable contributions in the areas of mass media and work with the youth. In addition, thousands of secondary school teachers were trained in life skills and HIV/AIDS and large amounts of materials were purchased to supply the schools.

AIDS activists have been vocal in defence of human rights and campaigning for access to treatment. They have been ably supported by academic and legal institutions such as the AIDS Law Project of the Centre for Applied Legal Studies at the University of the Witwatersrand, and Lawyers for Human Rights. The National Association of People with AIDS (NAPWA) has been a lobby for those most immediately affected by the disease. Together, these organisations and individuals have proven to be a capable watchdog of government and business activities. More than this, they are part of the fabric of the civil society in which the hope of stemming the epidemic must be vested.

The AIDS Directorate recognised that the levels of awareness around AIDS were high and so developed the Beyond Awareness communication campaigns. The basis for these campaigns was that most people had gained enough knowledge about HIV and AIDS and how to protect themselves; but they did not see *themselves* as being at risk. The question was how to go beyond knowledge to action. The Beyond Awareness campaign took the debate to a more personal level, encouraging people to confront their vulnerability, and linking them to resources such as the AIDS helpline operated by Life Line.

National STD management protocols were adopted, based on the syndromic approach. The latter recognises categories of STDs and treats them as such, rather than trying to identify any one specific STD which requires sophisticated laboratory back-up. The STD programme remains one of the pillars of the National AIDS Programme with efforts to ensure consistent supplies of drugs, the promotion of awareness and health-seeking activities, and training in both the public and private sectors.

Extensive training of service providers and managers in the public health sector was conducted. Access to barrier methods, primarily male condoms, was greatly improved despite ongoing problems with quality control. Over 150 million condoms were distributed free in 1999.

One of the major successes has been the introduction of annual surveillances to which we have already referred. Every year since 1990, in October and November, an anonymous survey of HIV prevalence has been conducted amongst pregnant women attending public health sector clinics. The results of these surveys, with careful interpretation, have provided a good indication of the progress of the epidemic in the general South African population. However, this knowledge has yet to be turned into concerted action. At the moment, we can be compared to a sinking ship having the ability to measure the water level on board down to the last millimetre; but we haven't got enough people manning the pumps to stop it slowly slipping beneath the waves!

MYTH
The country has done nothing so far in the fight against HIV and AIDS, and therefore deserves an 'E' rating.

REALITY
South Africa gets a 'C+' and a report card that reads: 'While some of the work has been good, it has been spoiled by careless mistakes. With a little more application and commitment, the country could do much better.'

Current position

As South Africa enters the new millennium and approaches a third decade of the AIDS epidemic, the government is clearly serious about addressing the epidemic. Media coverage is extensive and progressively more responsible. Efforts to destigmatise AIDS and ensure meaningful participation of people living with HIV and AIDS continue and the human rights lobby remains very active. A new HIV/AIDS Strategic Plan for 2000-2005, which draws on the strengths of the NACOSA plan, emphasises an intersectoral response, and this is slowly emerging. Traditional healers and trade unions are amongst the partners who have made most progress in defining their roles and commencing implementation.

Various forums have been established to facilitate the formation and operation of partnerships, notably the National AIDS Council which was launched early in 2000 and is chaired by the Deputy President, Jacob Zuma. This fills the gap left by the disbanding of the AIDS Advisory Committee which consisted of technical experts to advise on national AIDS programmes. The new council is perhaps the most concerted effort to date to bring together sectoral representatives. It will be supported by an international panel of experts who, apart from looking at 'the science of AIDS', will generally assist in policy formulation. Other forums include the Civil Military Alliance Against AIDS and the Interdepartmental Committee made up of representatives from various national government departments. The South African Business Council on HIV/AIDS (SABCOHA) has been relaunched with the intention that companies form a united front to fight AIDS in the workplace. The common purpose running through all these bodies is to encourage co-ordination; to exchange experiences and information about new developments and best practice; and to share resources. The Minister of Health has met with traditional leaders, faith-based organisations and the media to ensure their participation too.

A welcome development is that top businessman Bongani Khumalo has been appointed to head a powerful new anti-HIV/AIDS and rural development directorate in the President's office. He will report directly to Deputy President Jacob Zuma. His main role is expected to be the co-ordination of the government's efforts to fight the epidemic as well as the healing of the state's relationship with NGOs.

Case study: the KwaZulu-Natal (KZN) Cabinet initiative

In KZN, there is a provincial Cabinet initiative against AIDS, with political commitment at the highest level. A new provincial strategy to combat and manage the AIDS epidemic was announced by the Premier, Lionel Mtshali, on 29 October 1999 and ratified shortly afterwards by the KZN Cabinet. AIDS Challenge 2000 is a programme of action aimed at reducing the rate and level of HIV/AIDS infection in KZN with the ultimate aim of creating an AIDS-free society within a generation (the next 15 to 25 years). To achieve this aim, the KZN Cabinet has committed an annual amount of R20 million, starting from the 2001 financial year, to provide a platform for joint action against the spread of HIV/AIDS by all persons in society.

An additional amount of R1,4 million per year for staffing of a special Provincial HIV/AIDS Action Unit is being made available as from 2000. In conjunction with this initiative, a project aimed at making the already established AIDS pandemic in the province manageable and minimising its negative effects on development is getting off the ground. At the centre of all these programmes will be a communication campaign resting on several pillars:

■ the effective co-ordination of government departments and other role players in an overall information drive;
■ the use of the mainstream media to assist in the drive;
■ the mass mobilisation of people at grassroots level; and
■ the destigmatisation of HIV in all communities, together with the message that being open about the disease will reduce the rate of new infections.

Other initiatives

The life-skills programme has been extended into selected primary schools. Parallel to this, a youth programme has been established which targets youth through informal social mechanisms and youth organisations.

The On the Right Track AIDS train, which is in effect a moving AIDS conference, travelled around the country in 1999 featuring discussions on AIDS. The meetings included delegates from government, women's organisations and the media. Phase two will highlight issues involving women and AIDS, soliciting information from

women about their concerns and asking them for recommendations. The aim is to mobilise and organise women from all walks of
life to fight AIDS.

A new project aimed at containing HIV/AIDS in the road freight
industry was recently launched. Trucking Against AIDS is a joint
project of the Transport Department, trade unions and the road
freight industry (including Engen, Mercedes-Benz and the Road
Transport Industry Education and Training Board).

At the provincial level, Gauteng's provincial directors have
recognised the scale of the problem and the need for responses.
The provincial Department of Health was allocated additional resources and attempts have been made to plan for AIDS and HIV
prevention across all functions of provincial government.

Nationwide, local government – the level of government closest
to the people and with constitutional obligations to promote social
and economic development and to work with marginalised groups –
has, until recently, been slow to accept its responsibility as it relates
to AIDS. A toolkit, containing the tools which local governments
require to develop their response to AIDS, has been field-tested in
KZN with encouraging results. A second toolkit targets government
at the national level, particularly Departments such as Education,
Finance, Housing and Health which have very specific responsibilities in respect of AIDS.[2]

Developmental NGOs have been recognised as potentially important partners, situated in communities as they are with established infrastructures and credibility. Training has been conducted to
equip personnel from these NGOs with the skills and knowledge
necessary to take on AIDS issues.

Bristol-Myers Squibb, the pharmaceutical company, recently
launched their Secure the Future initiative which makes available
$100 million for five southern African countries over the next five
years. Much of the funding is earmarked for research which will
benefit women and children. Other ongoing research focuses on
mother-to-child transmission. Vaccine research, co-funded by
donors like the World Bank and led by the South African AIDS
Vaccine Initiative, remains the long-term hope for the future.

The announcement by Pfizer, another pharmaceutical company,

that it would provide Diflucan at no charge to AIDS patients in South Africa with cryptococcal meningitis is commendable. A single dose normally costs between R60 and R88 a day.[3] This has been followed by an announcement by five of the world's largest pharmaceutical companies – Bristol Myers Squibb and Merck of the US, Germany's Boehringer-Ingelheim, UK-based Glaxo Wellcome and Switzerland's Hoffman La Roche – that they are ready to investigate ways of lowering the prices of their HIV/AIDS drugs for African and other developing nations. Glaxo Wellcome, for example, has specifically offered Combivir – a combination of its antiretroviral drugs AZT and 3TC – at around $2 for a daily dose compared with $16,50 that it charges in the US.[4] Provisos to any new arrangement are that:

■ it only applies to drugs bought by government for public sector use;

■ drug companies may deal with countries on a case-by-case basis; and

■ the drugs have to be safely and effectively administered and their distribution controlled.

The last proviso is important because, in the absence of a proper distribution network, compliance may be patchy. This in turn could lead to resistant strains of HIV spreading among the population, making the situation even worse. Furthermore, the final details of the offer are not yet known and, as we all know, the devil is in the detail.

The problem of increasing numbers of children who have been or will be orphaned by AIDS is receiving attention at the highest levels. The following elements have been identified as priorities in preparing for all these orphans:[5]

■ policies are developed which assign responsibilities for the orphans at national, provincial and local government level;

■ communities are mobilised into providing facilities where necessary;

■ the issue of orphans is inserted into all programmes designed to alleviate poverty; and

■ a comprehensive database of orphans is kept.

The Metropolitan Group has launched an AIDS information website, *www.redribbon.com*, for Africa. It is just one of the many attempts to raise awareness and create an environment for effective prevention. These sorts of initiatives complement the mass/multimedia campaigns such as Beyond Awareness and Soul City.

Migrancy has been a way of life in southern Africa for decades. Now there are a number of bold initiatives by the mining industry to address the factors which lead to an increased risk of HIV transmission. For example, several mines are working closely with their neighbouring communities to establish credible campaigns to halt the spread of HIV; and more recently, they have extended these campaigns to the places where mine workers come from and to which they are repatriated when they have terminal AIDS.

Bridges have been built with other countries which have had to cope with the epidemic. Uganda was visited by a top-level South African delegation in 1999. In recognition of the fact that AIDS does not respect political or geographical boundaries, cross-border interventions are presently being planned along the major transport arteries, e.g. Durban-Lusaka.

NGOs and other organisations are developing treatment guidelines and models of community/home-based care including curricula for caregivers. The AIDS Unit at the University of Pretoria has put together a comprehensive package which could transform the response to the epidemic. It includes:
- the production of home-based care kits;
- the education of home-based carers and buddy teams;
- development of guidelines for nutrition;
- an understanding of the legal process of illness and death in terms of access to health care, creation of wills and plans for dependants; and
- community participation and education.

Dedicated community health workers provide excellent care and support to hundreds of HIV-infected clients in their homes. Critical though their work is, all the people on the ground are reporting increasing pressure on their services, and all admit that there are vast areas where no NGOs exist and no services are possible. The

131

fact that, on a daily basis, dozens of families in these areas are being precipitated into a crisis will one day have to be recognised.

AIDS and the future of government

As has been stated, but it bears repeating, AIDS causes increased morbidity and mortality among adults in the prime of their life. Many of the economic and social impacts were explored in previous chapters. Here, we will look at the consequences for government and hence the nation:

■ Society will lose a substantial fraction of the people who currently keep the wheels of commerce and the state turning, and from whose ranks the next generation of leaders will emerge.

■ The reservoir of national *human capital* will be depleted. The people who die will have had resources invested in them – they will have completed their education and training and will have accumulated valuable experience. Their death means that this investment is lost.

■ Social instability will rise in the absence of clear political leadership. In societies facing economic crisis and lacking clear political leadership, the presence of AIDS with its associated stigma can cause a revolution with many unwelcome aspects. *Somebody will be blamed.* On the other hand, the nation could settle into a state of listlessness, denial and anomie as it slides into oblivion.

■ The United States National Intelligence Council of the Central Intelligence Agency warns that 'the relationship between disease and political instability is indirect but real'; and that the infectious disease burden will weaken the military capabilities of some countries, with the cost being highest among the officers and the more modernised military forces in sub-Saharan Africa.[6]

■ There is a danger of human rights being infringed. Such infringement could even be entrenched in the legal system, if actions such as making AIDS notifiable are not thought through properly.

■ Government inefficiency is likely to result from the fact that government tends to have generous conditions of employment and operates in a less flexible fashion. Thus, it is quite possible that people who fall ill will have extended periods of sick leave during which their posts will not be filled and their work will not be done.

■ Orphans will represent a long-term threat to stability and development unless there are imaginative efforts to address the problem.

However, if AIDS is going to affect government, then the converse is also true. The style and type of government will affect both the spread of HIV and the impact that AIDS will have. The biomedical lobby looks at factors such as the behaviour patterns in society, use of condoms, the virus subtype and the existence of STDs to determine the speed of the spread of HIV. In reality, the causes are far more complex. As was discussed in Chapter 5, two concepts are crucial to understanding a society's susceptibility and vulnerability to HIV and AIDS:

- the degree of social cohesion in society; and
- the overall level of wealth.

The significance of this is simple. Countries with a highly developed civil society and good governance are less likely to experience an HIV epidemic than those without these characteristics. Indeed, it is possible that the response in Uganda has been relatively successful because it is attempting to build a civil society at the same time as it is responding to the epidemic. This message needs to be carried over into the final chapter when we look at the challenge for South Africa. We will find it much easier to find ways of responding to the epidemic that work and make a difference if our initiatives are accompanied by moves to promote a civil society.

10 The challenge of AIDS for South Africa

AIDS is the greatest challenge facing South Africa, something which is increasingly being recognised. As mentioned in the previous chapter, there is evidence that the political leadership is aware of the enormity of the problem and will devote greater energy to overcoming it. For example, President Mbeki wrote in a letter[1] to President Clinton dated 3 April 2000: 'In 1998, our government decided radically to step up its own efforts to combat AIDS, this fight having, up to this point, been left largely to our Ministry and Department of Health.'

We have experienced a quantum increase in press coverage since the famous occasion when a national daily chose to run with what Monica Lewinsky said to Barbara Walters as its headline story, whilst consigning the latest antenatal clinic data to page three. There are no longer *any* South Africans who do not know someone or of someone who has died of AIDS or is living with HIV. In many of the townships at weekends, instead of parties and weddings, people attend funerals. The red AIDS ribbon which adorns the cover of this book is seen everywhere; it is almost *de rigueur* to wear it if you classify yourself as a new South African.

The key priorities

But what are our priorities? How can we meet the challenge? A number of key points need to be made by way of introduction to this chapter:

■ *There is no easy answer, no quick fix, no magic bullet.* Pinning one's hopes on a vaccine or cure is an unsound strategy at this stage. If either is discovered, it's a windfall. Hence, sitting back and waiting for a breakthrough is as bad as basing the management of your personal finances on winning the lottery! The more realistic scenario is that the medical fraternity will develop treatment regimes which are simpler to administer and cheaper to use and

134

which turn HIV into a chronic but manageable ailment. This will take time and time is not on our side.

■ *The little things will make a difference.* In concluding this book, we are not about to offer a revolutionary new vision or formula for fighting the epidemic. The days of marching to the drum of some monolithic global AIDS strategy are gone. It's about doing lots of little things better at grassroots level, with the emphasis on *doing*. There are so many community and NGO initiatives worth building on and intensifying. One must not underestimate the therapeutic value of working together in small groups – where everybody is in the same boat – to overcome a problem. Moreover, nobody knows what the best responses are and it is only by trying them all out that we can start honing in on the ones showing the optimum results.

■ *Everyone has a role to play.* This epidemic is only going to be conquered when the population as a whole is mobilised against it. If HIV had been a human enemy on our border threatening to kill a quarter of the population, we could appeal to people's patriotism to serve on the front and repel the enemy. In HIV's case, the front is in everyone's home. But the virus is fragile and can be beaten.

■ *We need leadership.* In countries like Uganda and Thailand, the epidemic is being turned around by highly visible political leadership. Not a day goes by without exhortations by the leaders on radio and TV and in visits to every part of the country to fight HIV. We need people of the calibre of Mbeki and Mandela to be out on the hustings and in the school halls, fighting the campaign of their lives.

As President Mbeki said in another excerpt from the letter quoted above: 'It is obvious that whatever lessons we have to and may draw from the West about the grave issue of HIV-AIDS, a simple superimposition of Western experience on African reality would be absurd and illogical. Such proceedings would constitute a criminal betrayal of our responsibility to our people.' We agree with the sentiment that an African solution must be found to AIDS in Africa. But we also believe that HIV causes AIDS and Western therapies, at affordable prices, should be an integral part of our arsenal in the war against the virus.

Acknowledgement of past failures

Despite the cautious optimism we must all feel from the latest antenatal clinic data, we must still acknowledge our failures in preventing the spread of HIV and learn from them. We have certainly shown little ability in responding to the rising tide of AIDS cases. In part, the blame for this must be laid at the way we have responded to the epidemic. The response has gone through three stages:

Stage 1. *It is not our problem.* To begin with, we set out to convince people that AIDS was a problem. This was done through giving data and projections. But we did not show people that it was *their problem*. The result was that white people saw it as a black problem; black people saw it as a gay white problem; and rich people saw it as a problem of the poor (and in many cases still do). Worse still, given that there was no real evidence of AIDS cases, no one really believed it was a problem anyway.

Stage 2. *We have a problem.* The next step was to show that the problem was one we all needed to take on board – i.e. it was *our problem*. Again, this had to be done through projections rather than hard data – but we were able to draw examples from countries to the north. This stage of advocacy was helped by the fact that the reality of AIDS was beginning to be felt. However, we did not present any solutions. Thus, we were warning that the train was coming down the tracks but were not saying what we could do to stop or divert it. This was *disempowering* and resulted in people and leaders feeling helpless and thus avoiding the issue. This can be illustrated by reference to another global issue – global warming and climate change. Few South Africans would argue that our weather patterns are unchanged: floods, heat waves and droughts seem increasingly common and severe. Most suspect that global warming is contributing to this and believe something should be done, but don't know what *they* can do.

Stage 3. *We have a problem and we can deal with it.* This is the stage which we are now coming to in South Africa and on which we need

136

to consolidate our efforts. There is a problem but there are things we can do individually and collectively. This has been the theme of our book all along and calls for extensive networking. Consequently, we have included as Appendix 3 a list of useful contacts. But this is only the start. We need a significant initiative – orchestrated perhaps by the insurance industry in the private sector – to publicise in each and every community the places where people should go to obtain detailed information on HIV/AIDS.

MYTH
HIV/AIDS is somebody else's problem, not mine.
REALITY
Somehow or somewhere the epidemic will intrude on all our lives, and a selfish attitude will only make matters worse.

In formulating our response to the challenge, two broad areas of priorities exist:
■ Prevention; and
■ Dealing with the impact.

Prevention
Preventing new infections must remain first prize. It is more cost-effective than treatment. Chart 10.1 shows just how much the course of the epidemic can be changed if the interventions mentioned in it are successful. It supports the key messages of this book which are:
■ Even in the worst affected provinces where up to 30 per cent of adults may be infected, this means that 70 per cent are not.
■ In those parts of South Africa where HIV prevalence is comparatively low, the challenge is to keep it so.
■ Each year a new cohort of young people are growing to adulthood and sexual activity. They can, and should, be kept HIV-free.

Identifying prevention as a goal is the easy part. Now comes the difficult part: deciding what to do. The first lesson is that we need to focus our activities by age group and even by province. The second lesson is to accept that much of what has been done so far is highly appropriate and these activities should be further supported. They fall into three types:

Knowledge and education. Most adults are sufficiently aware of AIDS. The next step is to move beyond awareness, and this is a priority of the government. There are two crucial areas where more is needed. Firstly, schools need to be used for AIDS education and the programme should start at a very early age – probably when a child is six years old. We feel that the programme should be aimed at teaching life skills rather than focusing on HIV and AIDS alone. A similar technique has been used successfully to warn children of the dangers of drug abuse. In addition, parents need to take some responsibility for this education. However hard it is to broach the subject, parents should remember that it is the lives of their children that are at stake. It's no longer the case of teaching about the birds and bees just to prevent unwanted pregnancies!

But there are others who should be involved in spelling out the message. Evidence suggests that a critical factor for successful prevention is leadership. Leaders at all levels, from the President to the village headman or councillor, from the preacher in the pulpit to the captain of industry at a school prize-giving, from sports heroes to soap opera stars, should be taking every opportunity to talk about HIV and lead by example.

At present, we believe that the majority of South Africans do not really understand the epidemic or its nuances and subtleties. People need to appreciate for example the difference between HIV and AIDS, the scale of the problem and the future trends with and without positive interventions.

Condoms and other barriers to infection. Condoms should be readily available, affordable and of acceptable quality. These issues are increasingly being addressed. What is not being looked at is their acceptability. A very simple point is that condoms are all made of white latex. According to research carried out in Gauteng: 'Black teenagers and young adults unanimously state that they do not like the "white" condoms. Why do they have to wear "white" condoms? It looks stupid. All subjects said that condoms are boring and clinical, including the packaging. They want different colours, even scented condoms. They would use more condoms if they were more fun.'[2] Has anyone thought of doing a market survey on the most attractive colour for condoms for black and white teenagers? It would not be expensive.

Use of male condoms requires the assent of the male partner. There is an urgent need, therefore, to improve female condoms and look at other prevention methods. Here, microbicides are crucial as they kill the virus in the vagina and can be inserted by a woman without her partner's awareness and hence permission. This is being researched in South Africa.

Chart 10.1   Impacts of preventive measures (*introduced over 2000 to 2005*)[3]

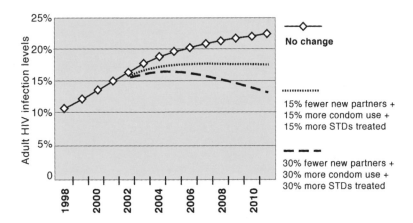

STD treatment. The early and correct treatment of STDs is an important weapon in the armoury against HIV transmission. It needs further attention. Encouraging women in particular to seek proper reproductive health care should be a priority, as they often don't know there is something wrong with them or are prepared to live with a problem – seeing it as part of a woman's lot in life. Even when they do seek care they are still likely to get an incorrect diagnosis and/or treatment.

It is clear that while these existing activities have been *necessary,* they have not been *sufficient*. Other new interventions are also required. For example, voluntary testing followed by counselling has largely been ignored. Yet, if people don't know that they are HIV positive, they cannot make the decision as to whether or not to risk infecting other people. Moreover, if people decide to be tested and discover they are HIV negative, then they will have an incentive to remain that way. The key is the quality and availability of testing and counselling.

Other interventions. A potentially fruitful area is to look upstream at what can be done to change the environment in which people live and make decisions about their sexual behaviour. Essentially, the goal is to empower people so that they can make decisions which will reduce risk of infection. This means examining the socio-economic causes of the epidemic and countering them. Here are certain priorities:

■ Although much has been done, the migrant labour system is still fuelling the epidemic and ensuring that HIV reaches into all communities in southern Africa. Government and private sector employers should ensure that migrants have the opportunity and ability to bring their families to live with them at their place of work. More housing and land may have to be made available to achieve this objective.

■ Actions to enhance the status of women are crucial. These range from giving them training and capital to become entrepreneurs to tougher laws on rape and sexual harassment.

■ Children, and particularly orphans, are vulnerable to sexual molestation. This subject must be given a proper airing and measures instituted to bring up all children in a caring environment.

■ Home ownership and electrification should be pursued. Work elsewhere in Africa finds that home-owners are less likely to be infected because they have a long-term perspective and avoid risky behaviour. Electrification automatically raises people's standard of living and gives them access to a whole range of recreational activities.

Building a civil society is essential so that all sectors of South African society can respond to the threat of HIV in an imaginative way. However, this is not something that can be imposed by the state, but rather has to evolve with the state's encouragement. We also believe that there should be far greater involvement of people living with HIV/AIDS in all aspects of the response. But we recognise that this can only happen if the disease is destigmatised and a caring environment is created. We could go on adding to the list of preventive measures. Much better, though, is for you, the reader, to look at what you do in your professional and personal life and ask what you can do to protect yourself and those who work for and with you.

Dealing with the impact

The lack of success of prevention means that South Africa has to deal with the impact flowing from the illness and death of large numbers of people. We have shown that this will be on a scale in excess of anything experienced to date. One of the main problems around the epidemic is having people conceive of the size of the problem and sadly its inevitability. Those who will fall ill and die during the course of the next few years are already infected. Thus, the future of South Africa will to a large extent be determined by how quickly the penny drops that the impact of AIDS has to be dealt with.

AIDS will initially be felt by the health sector as the number of people needing care begins to rise. Already a significant percentage of South Africa's public sector hospital beds are occupied by those with HIV-related illnesses. This proportion is set to rise in the years ahead. The private sector provides health care for a sizeable percentage of South Africans, most of whom are covered through medical aid schemes. The total covered at the end of 1999 was estimated at around 7,5 million, including family dependants.[4] However, the schemes have ceilings on the amount of care they will fund, and sometimes only provide cover for people while they are in employment. Those people whose medical aid cover lapses when they are too ill to work will be forced to seek care in the public sector. This will add to an already stretched situation.

One of the principal challenges for the private sector is to understand the benefits in providing care for their workers. As Appendix 1 shows, there are a number of treatment regimes that can prolong the healthy and productive lives of the workforce. In one of the three schemes mentioned, 1 935 patients have been on the programme for two years or more, of which 31 have been hospitalised and 18 have died. In the absence of treatment, it is estimated that at least half of the total number would have been hospitalised or died.[5]

In addition, we anticipate that the cost of drugs will come down over the next few years. Abt Associates South Africa Inc. in its excellent document *The Impending Catastrophe: A Resource Book on the Emerging HIV/AIDS Epidemic in South Africa* has this to say on current treatment costs: "For triple anti-retroviral therapy to at least pay for itself through savings in other HIV-related health costs, it would have to cost less than one tenth of current market prices in South Africa . . . such drastic price reductions seem unlikely." This may be so, but the latest announcements by international drug companies mean that we 'might be on our way to meeting that objective. Moreover, as we highlighted in Chapter 8, if you take into account all the other costs associated with HIV/AIDS sickness and death, the cost to a company of giving its HIV-positive employees treatment is probably less now than the cost of not doing so (apart from which the employees concerned will be less infectious). Of course, all this raises a number of thorny questions:

■ In what circumstances can testing legally and morally be undertaken? It is hoped that clear guidelines which take into account the interests of all parties will be established soon.

■ Should South Africa seek to manufacture cheaper generic equivalents locally or to import them in parallel? In answering this question, one has to bear in mind the difficulty of quality control for generic drugs, especially if they are imported.

■ How does one stop round-tripping whereby antiretroviral drugs are purchased locally at deep discounts and marketed back into America and Europe?

■ Should South Africa allow in HIV patients from other countries in Africa to receive treatment if it is not available to them in their home country? If not, how does South Africa stop illegal immigrants coming in for treatment?

The challenge for the public sector is rather different. It must provide appropriate treatment within the constraints of a limited budget. HIV/AIDS will be the single biggest health care issue for years to come. Limits on resources for health care, and massively increased need, mean that HIV/AIDS must be fully integrated into all aspects of welfare and health-care planning. Failure to do this will result in injustice to people with HIV/AIDS and people with other health needs.

In the near future, the public sector will have to undertake two exercises:

■ to assess whether money can be switched from other areas of government to augment health-care expenditure;

■ to plan a health-care delivery system which meets HIV/AIDS needs in an affordable and cost-effective way.

The latter exercise is not something that can be left to doctors who are ethically bound to seek the best care for patients regardless of cost. It will require the input of professional hospital administrators who are used to balancing patient needs against available funds.

One of the ways to relieve some of the pressure will be to provide home-based care for patients who cannot benefit from hospital care. Home-based care can be most cost-effective and will increasingly be invoked as the hospitals fill up. It will need careful planning and support to the families if it is not to turn into home-based neglect. As already mentioned, the University of Pretoria's Centre for the Study of AIDS has identified this as a key area and has developed a 'home-care kit'. For many families, the prime need will be food and clothing. If they don't have these, talk of providing care is pointless. Care is a 'continuum' from catering for elementary needs to raising the quality of life and psychological state of the recipient. This is as true for a family as it is for an infected person.

Apart from care, affected families may need support in many other forms. If we expect families to bear the burden of AIDS illnesses and death, then they may have to be given a grant in cash or kind. This will go against the grain of moving away from direct hand-outs, but it will be extremely difficult for a relatively wealthy country like South Africa to walk away from such an obligation.

Of particular concern is the impact of AIDS on children. Writing in *AIDS Analysis Africa,* Stephen Morgan, who is the South African Director of Save the Children Fund (UK) in South Africa, argues that while we must 'take full cognisance of the consequences of a rapidly increasing orphan population . . . it is, however, both dangerous and wrong to exclude the very real needs and rights of other children, all of whom will be affected by the pandemic . . . A recent study commissioned by the National HIV/AIDS Care & Support Task Team in South Africa,[6] and funded by Save the Children Fund (UK), identifies a variety of categories when defining *Children living with HIV/AIDS.* Amongst the most threatened groups identified were those children from "infected" households who are affected in a range of ways both before and after the deaths of their parents. This clearly incorporates orphans but also includes those children who live in families where parents are still alive but who may be periodically ill. These children have to assume similar responsibilities to those of orphans, coupled with the additional burden of caring for their dying parents. Responses to HIV/AIDS need to incorporate planning for the future of children who will be orphaned, as well as providing support for those children who act as caregivers whilst their parents are still alive'.[7]

The consequences of *not* caring for the affected children will be felt throughout society for many generations to come. To avert this social disaster will again call for an imaginative response and it will have to come from both the public and private sectors working in partnership. One suggestion is to train surrogate parents selected by communities and church groups in conjunction with local authorities. Orphans (and here no distinction should be drawn between AIDS and non-AIDS orphans) will be housed with their surrogate parents who will be paid a small salary for supervision and be provided with sufficient funds to cover food, clothing and incidental expenses. The system, which could be operated through the Department of Welfare, will require monitoring. NGOs might be the appropriate bodies to do this. The costs in aggregate of implementing such a proposal may be high, but the costs of not doing it – and producing a generation of neglected young men and women – will be even higher. Moreover, it highlights the point that the extra resources required to cope with the AIDS epidemic are not just monetary. It will need human resources as well. The horrible irony is that these resources will be depleted by the epidemic at the very time they are most needed.

While on the subject of children, we would be remiss in not pointing out the impact of AIDS on the education system. It is sad that, just as the South African education system is coming out of crisis, AIDS will mean fewer teachers, planners and administrators. Yet, weeks of education lost from children's lives can never be replaced; special tuition and care will be needed for children who are orphaned or infected themselves; and the education system is where prevention must begin. So it is a matter of the highest priority to have an educational plan in place which specifically copes with the consequences of the epidemic.

Conclusion

The AIDS challenge is enormous. But people must not feel powerless. It is all about action on many different fronts. Before this battle is over, there will be many ordinary people who will become heroes and heroines in their own communities. Perhaps we will learn to care more for each other and exercise more responsibility in our sexual behaviour. Perhaps we will learn the true meaning of being a rainbow nation. Perhaps we will create that civil society we all yearn for.

At the XIIIth International AIDS Conference held in Durban in July 2000, the theme was 'Break the Silence'. It was not only an acknowledgement of the many silences which surround and imprison HIV/AIDS, but an invitation to the global community to have open debates, to discover new facts and to share experiences. We hope that, by writing this book, we will stimulate South Africans to feel a similar sense of freedom in honestly discussing the implications of HIV/AIDS for our society and the appropriate responses. We don't have all the answers. We don't pretend to. It would be quite at variance with the spirit of this book to make it sound like a comprehensive manual. We want you to dream up your own solutions and put them into practice. Some will be right, some will be wrong. But all will further the cause.

South Africa is a unique country. We have stared disaster in the face at a number of points in our recent history. But we've always managed to overcome the obstacles and move forward. AIDS presents another challenge: to expose the proposition that the disease is unstoppable, untreatable and undefeatable for what it is – *a total myth*. The reality is that every little thing counts. If we all put our shoulders to the wheel in our own ways, we can beat the bug. For our children's sake, let us not be found wanting!

Appendix 1 Treatment options

Mother-to-child transmission (MTCT)

Medical background[1]

A growing amount of research has been conducted into the cause and possible prevention of MTCT, with a number of important results. A child can be infected with HIV prenatally, at the time of delivery or postnatally through breast-feeding. Infection at delivery is the most common, leading to the practice of caesarean section as a method of reducing the risk of HIV infection. A number of factors influence the risk of transmission, particularly the viral load of the mother at birth – the higher the load, the higher the risk. Another factor affecting the risk of MTCT is the type of the mother's virus: rapid/high virus isolates are associated with transmission and slow/low virus isolates are associated with nontransmission. A low CD4 count is also associated with increased risk. Antiretroviral drugs may decrease the viral load and inhibit viral reproduction in the infant, thus decreasing the risk of MTCT. To test this hypothesis, the AIDS Clinical Trial Group conducted a study at a number of sites in the US. The study involved administering AZT to HIV-positive pregnant women in 100 mg dosages five times a day from 14-34 weeks (with a median of 26 weeks) of pregnancy until delivery. An additional oral dose of AZT was given to the infant. All women in the trial had CD4 counts above 200, were symptom-free and had not taken AZT before. The results of the trial showed a 67,5 per cent reduction in transmission. The high cost of the course ($1 500 or R10 500 per mother-child pair) and the complexity of adhering to it have meant that only the richer nations are using this intervention at the moment.

The search for cheaper and simpler alternatives has led to a number of trials of short-course antiretroviral drugs. The greater risk of transmission in the later stages of pregnancy and during delivery means that a shorter treatment period produces only a small reduction in efficiency. In addition, it lessens the risk of noncompliance associated with long-term courses. The Centres for Disease Control sponsored a trial of short-course AZT in Thailand, involving the administering of AZT for the last four weeks of pregnancy. The results showed a 50 per cent reduction in transmission. Similarly, the PETRA (Perinatal Transmission) study undertaken in five urban settings in South Africa, Uganda and Tanzania showed transmission reductions of between 37 and 50 per cent, depending on whether children were breast-fed or not. In Uganda, trials involving short-course dosages of nevirapine also produced a 50 per cent reduction in MTCT.

Costs

The cost of providing long-course antiretroviral treatment is prohibitively expensive for the poorer nations. Even with the 75 per cent reduction in AZT's price offered by Glaxo Wellcome, the drugs alone cost more than $200 per mother-baby pair.[2] The short-course Thai and PETRA regimens are, however, significantly cheaper at around $89 for the drugs. The cost of nevirapine for each treatment in the Ugandan regimen is even lower at $4.[3] However, these costs are not the only ones requiring consideration. Counselling and testing cost approximately $7 per person.[4] Six months of formula feed amounts to $60 per person.

The cost of the aforementioned regimens in the South African context has been reported by Mascolini.[5] The long course of AZT would cost R1 562 per mother-child pair, the short course with AZT R562 and the short course with nevirapine R35. However, the avoidance of expensive hospitalisation charges could mean that a short course of either AZT or nevirapine may save on costs in a South African setting.[6 and 7]

Nevirapine is still under consideration by the Medicines Control Council in South Africa. Although reports say that the council has approved the drug, the body is still reviewing data from Uganda where the drug has been tested. The Department of Health said that a decision on whether the government would buy the drug for use in its hospitals and clinics would be made only when all the relevant test information from local drug trials was available.

Disease management schemes

The second part of this appendix outlines three programmes that are currently available in South Africa to treat people living with HIV and AIDS.

LifeSense Disease Management

LifeSense offers products to medical schemes and companies aimed at providing a complete and holistic management programme for dealing with HIV and AIDS.

Innovative and recognised long-term suppressive treatments are implemented to reduce workplace absenteeism and HIV patients' hospitalisation periods, while increasing a patient's projected life span. Costs to the company's medical scheme, or member, are kept at affordable levels. Specifically, the programme incorporates clinical treatment protocols and data to assess risk and to enable future planning. HIV-positive members are able to access up-to-date and effective medical care; they are encouraged to take responsibility for their own wellbeing; and they are assisted with dietary require-ments and exercise programmes.

LifeSense offers a confidential call centre during office hours and is staffed by skilled and qualified personnel. This call centre is able to assist patients and their dependants with counselling and in-formation regarding the enrolment process. A nurse is assigned to a medical scheme and is responsible for the ongoing training of case managers and assisting with the identification of members and their enrolment. Clinical consultants are contracted to develop sustain-able treatment protocols for clients.

To date, this service has been provided to a number of medical reimbursement companies that cover approximately one million lives. All attempts are made to align treatment costs with the re-imbursement limits set by the funder. Where this is not feasible, members are clearly informed that they may be required to make a reasonable co-payment.

The protocol content is formulated according to internationally accepted standards of care and adheres to the following principles:
■ Evidence-based efficacy from international clinical trials;

- Sustainability;
- Preservation of future treatment options;
- Patient acceptability;
- Cost-effective utilisation of laboratory investigations.

The products offered include a series of educational modules for education and training of staff together with a facilitator. The scope of the curriculum includes:

General HIV/AIDS education and awareness
- Presentation to management and employees;
- Distribution of educational literature;
- Dedicated LifeSense Disease Management consultant;
- Prearranged scheduling for ongoing education;
- Induction education for new employees.

Occupational medical personnel
- Core knowledge of the virology, epidemiology and diagnosis of HIV infection;
- Medical and immunological aspects of HIV disease;
- Concepts of antiretroviral therapy and opportunistic disease prophylaxis;
- Psychosocial aspects of HIV infection;
- Primary counselling skills for professional and lay persons;
- Developing and utilising community resources for HIV infection;
- Infection control and home nursing;
- HIV in the workplace;
- Legal, commercial and ethical aspects of HIV infection;
- Lifestyle management and wellness programmes.

LifeSense resources are also used to develop a capacity-building course to meet the specific needs of the client. The process usually involves a team leader from LifeSense Disease Management who works with small groups and individuals.

Cost structure

The cost of the risk management product varies from scheme to scheme. A monthly administration fee is charged according to the membership of the scheme and negotiations with the client. The management fee includes the initial application; precertification assessment; production of precertification forms and the provision of these to practitioners; the collation of data from the practitioners for review by a LifeSense Disease Management specialist; and the return of recommendations to the primary caregiver via the client. The monthly management fee also serves as payment for quarterly data review and ongoing clinical recommendations, whenever required, by LifeSense Disease Management clinical consultants.

The cost of the ongoing educational courses starts at R2 500 per month for employers with less than 300 employees up to a maximum of R5 000 per month for large employer groups.

Contact details:

Dr André van Bassen
LifeSense Disease Management
86 Oxford Road
Houghton Estates
2198
Tel: (011) 880 1884

Fax: (011) 880 4960/447 5841
Website: *www.lifesense.co.za*
PO Box 1774
Parklands
2121

Lifeworks

Lifeworks' Positivelife programme addresses the issue of HIV/AIDS and its management on an individualised but nationwide scale. Lifeworks states that, by harnessing existing professional expertise and making sound use of employee benefits and medical aid funds, it can medically manage all working people with HIV/AIDS within a company at less than one per cent of that company's payroll.

The importance of education in awareness and prevention is recognised but Positivelife's focus is on reducing the impact of HIV/AIDS – through the identification of infected individuals and the active treatment of each individual.

In order to achieve these two fundamentals, Positivelife:

- determines the prevalence of HIV infection within any group;
- assesses the projected risk of future infection within the group;
- identifies people with HIV infection within the group;
- treats the infected individuals; and
- treats all new infections within the group.

The outcome of this method of management of HIV/AIDS (or any other chronic illness) is a high percentage (80 per cent) of people remaining active or returning to the workplace. The rate of retaining people in the economy is further increased if the Positivelife programme is linked to Lifeworks' rehabilitation, reskilling and job placement of impaired people.

Lifeworks' Positivelife management of HIV/AIDS has a wide range of potential and actual clients. These include private sector employers, members of managed-care organisations, medical aid subscribers, trade union members, military personnel and civil servants. Whatever the size of the group, each case is treated individually by a network of specially trained privately practising doctors and HIV/AIDS counsellors. Countries covered include South Africa, Namibia, Swaziland, Botswana and Zimbabwe.

Each case is handled in private consulting facilities, on a stringently confidential, profoundly personal and holistic basis, for two reasons:
- Each HIV-infected person is an individual in his or her own right and is entitled to special care.
- Each individual has differing degrees of infection and may or may not have concomitant disease (such as opportunistic infection, malnutrition, etc.).

The programme has the following elements:
- Risk assessment and disease profile within any given group of people, utilising Lifeworks' AIDS Impact Calculator. This actuarial model identifies the probable prevalence in a group; projects the future incidence; and calculates the costs, the financial savings and the extension of productive life span consequent upon proper management of HIV/AIDS.
- Intensive and transparent education to help people realise the

advantages to be gained from voluntary and confidential submission to testing of a treatable disease by a network of privately practising counsellors and doctors.

■ Assessment of disease within individual companies through absentee monitoring (without notification to the employer of individual disease occurrences).

■ Individual, private and confidential counselling and treatment.

■ Redeployment, reskilling or placement with an alternative employer for people who are partially work-impaired by HIV/AIDS.

■ Lifelong medical management of each individual case.

Positivelife's philosophy is a simple one: HIV/AIDS is a manageable disease which can afflict anyone; and people with HIV/AIDS deserve affordable, personalised, effective and dignified treatment.

Contact details:

Dr Jack van Niftrik
Managing Director,
Lifeworks

Wayne Myslik
Head of Consulting Services,
Lifeworks

PO Box 41259
Craighall,
South Africa 2024
Tel: (011) 340 2632
Fax: (011) 880 8376
e-mail: *jniftrik@lifeworks.co.za*
wmyslik@lifeworks.co.za

Aid for AIDS

The Aid for AIDS programme aims to promote the early detection and treatment of HIV infection and to educate members of a medical scheme about the disease itself. In addition, the programme provides for access to antiretroviral therapy as well as the prevention and treatment of HIV/AIDS-related conditions within the budget of the scheme concerned. By providing access to these benefits, the progression of the disease can be slowed and the number of AIDS-related conditions and consequential hospitalisations can be reduced.

Aid for AIDS believes that the best way of improving the quality of life of members living with HIV/AIDS is not just by increasing the amount of money available, but also by offering a comprehensive disease-management programme. Hence the most appropriate treatment is selected in consultation with the responsible doctor. Thereafter, regular contact is maintained with both the doctor and patient. A full-time medical advisor is available to assist doctors with treatment queries. He is supported by a panel of expert HIV/AIDS clinicians who advise on complex problems.

As antiretroviral therapy must be carefully monitored to be effective and safe, regular blood tests are requested by Aid for AIDS and paid for by the medical scheme. The results are reviewed to ensure that the drugs are still effective and not causing harmful adverse effects. When necessary, the medical team contacts the doctor to update or amend therapy.

Regular advice is given to the members concerned on how the programme can help them, and on how to cope with HIV/AIDS. Other crucial issues, such as the importance of taking the correct treatment combination and not missing doses, are discussed. Any changes to the authorised therapy are also explained. This contact is made via the Aid for AIDS nurse-line, which is operated by experienced nursing consultants.

Aid for AIDS offers all pregnant women vertical (mother-to-child) transmission prevention. This includes AZT for the last four weeks of pregnancy, during delivery and to the baby for six weeks after delivery. In addition, caesarean section is facilitated as this reduces the risk of transmitting the virus. Milk substitutes will be funded for up to six months, as a substitute for breast-feeding. Babies are tested for HIV at six weeks.

Infected children may join the programme, and have access to all the benefits including antiretroviral therapy, where appropriate. A part-time paediatrician, who is an expert in the management of HIV-infected children, is available to assist the Aid for AIDS medical team.

If a member suffers a needle-stick injury or sexual assault, the Aid for AIDS programme provides postexposure prophylaxis with antiretroviral drugs.

The programme offers complete confidentiality. Employer groups and medical schemes have no access to the names of people on the programme. Aid for AIDS is situated in a restricted area with its own dedicated staff, all of whom have signed confidentiality agreements. The programme has its own communication and computer systems. Those staff involved with claims processing have also signed confidentiality agreements.

Hospitalisation is confidentially monitored as well to ensure that optimal use is made of different levels of care. This includes assisting people in an advanced AIDS condition to obtain additional help, such as step-down and hospice care.

Other benefits offered by Aid for AIDS include an education and awareness programme. Two trained professionals develop customised programmes for employer groups and medical scheme members, in order to improve employees' knowledge about HIV/AIDS and show them how to avoid becoming infected. Members living with HIV/AIDS are encouraged to join the programme at an early stage in order to assist with this education process, but also to have access to counselling and regular tests.

In addition, the medical staff of the programme participate in HIV/AIDS training programmes for doctors' groups throughout the country. These improve doctors' knowledge of the disease and advise them of the latest available treatment.

Currently, there are over 4 500 people registered with Aid for AIDS, many of whom are on antiretroviral therapy. The majority are responding well to treatment and feel the programme is of value to them.

There are 28 medical schemes contracted to Aid for AIDS, covering more than 1,5 million lives. The amount set aside for antiretroviral therapy varies according to the scheme, but is generally sufficient to cover the cost of at least dual therapy. Certain schemes will, however, cover the cost of triple therapy in full. Drug manufacturers have agreed to supply dispensing doctors and pharmacists at the best possible prices available. It should be stressed that members of contracted schemes and their dependants do not have to pay any additional money in order to join the programme.

Aid for AIDS ensures that members of contracted medical schemes and their dependants have access to reasonable ongoing benefits for HIV and AIDS within the framework of a comprehensive and confidential disease management programme. There is little doubt that HIV/AIDS should now be regarded as a manageable chronic disease, which can be treated cost-effectively; and in regard to MTCT prevented cost-effectively.

Contact Details:

Dr Leon Regensberg	Telephone:	Fax:
Aid for AIDS	(021) 658 6464	(021) 658 6426
Private Bag X1003	086 0100646	0800 600 773
Claremont		
7735		

Appendix 2 The legal framework and HIV/AIDS[1]

The way in which employees with HIV or AIDS are treated in the workplace has a multitude of legal implications. These extend from the highest level, the Constitution, right the way down to a shop-floor agreement between employer and employees. As with all law, its boundaries have to be tested through the courts – something that is starting to happen. Moreover, legislation and the way it is applied will continue to evolve to meet our changing knowledge and understanding of the epidemic.

The legislation

The South African Constitution (Act 108 of 1996) is the supreme law of the country and all other laws must comply with its provisions. The Bill of Rights within the Constitution sets out a number of rights which protects employees. As a result the government has, within the last five years, amended certain laws and introduced new pieces of legislation to ensure that our labour laws are consistent with the Constitution.

There are seven key pieces of labour legislation in South Africa, including one which applies specifically to the mining industry. These are:
- the Employment Equity Act No. 55 of 1998 (EEA);
- the Promotion of Equality and Prevention of Unfair Discrimination Act No. 4 of 2000;
- the Labour Relations Act No. 66 of 1995 (LRA);
- the Occupational Health and Safety Act No. 85 of 1993 (OHSA);
- the Mines Health and Safety Act No. 29 of 1996;
- the Compensation for Occupational Injuries and Diseases Act No. 130 of 1993 (COIDA); and
- the Basic Conditions of Employment Act No. 75 of 1997 (BCEA).

HIV/AIDS is only expressly referred to in the Employment Equity Act, but there are provisions in all the other Acts which have relevance to HIV/AIDS. The Employment Equity Act will, because of its express protection for employees against unfair discrimination on the basis of 'HIV status', become the most important point of reference for decisions relating to the management of HIV/AIDS in the workplace.[2]

There are also other pieces of legislation, policies and protections within the common law which, although not directly employment-related, impact on the management of HIV/AIDS in the workplace. These are:

■ the Medical Schemes Act No. 131 of 1998;
■ the proposed notification of AIDS disease and death;
■ the Department of Health's draft National Policy on Testing for HIV; and
■ common-law protection of the right to privacy and dignity.

South Africa has become a signatory to a number of international agreements and codes such as the International Labour Organisation (ILO) Convention 111 on Discrimination (Employment and Occupation), 1958. However, the only one which relates specifically to HIV/AIDS in the workplace is the Southern African Development Community (SADC) Code on AIDS and Employment which was approved by the Council of Ministers in September 1997. This Code provides a nondiscriminatory framework for managing HIV/AIDS in the workplace.

To provide an overview of the legal framework for employment relationships with a focus on those aspects which have HIV/AIDS implications, it is necessary to examine the relevant Constitutional provisions and the elements in the legislation which apply.

The Constitution and Employment Equity Acts

In the *Constitution Act No. 108 of 1996,* the Bill of Rights provides that every person has the right to equality and nondiscrimination (section 9), privacy (section 14), fair labour practices (section 23), and access to information (section 32). These rights are not absolute and may be limited provided such a limitation is reasonable and justifiable (section 36).

These rights should, in turn, be reflected in workplace policies and they should guide the nature and form of all employment relationships. In particular, the right to privacy implies an employee's right to confidentiality regarding medical information, including information about HIV status.

The *Employment Equity Act No. 55 of 1998* (EEA) aims at ensuring equality and nondiscrimination in the workplace through anti-discrimination measures and affirmative action (equality provisions). It also provides two express provisions on HIV/AIDS. Section 6(1) of the Act aims to promote equal opportunity by eliminating unfair discrimination and in addition prohibits unfair discrimination, directly or indirectly, against an employee in any employment policy or practice, on one or more grounds, including race, gender, sex, pregnancy, marital status, family responsibility, ethnic or social origin, colour, sexual orientation, age, disability, religion, HIV status, conscience, belief, political opinion, culture, language and birth.

Section 7 of the Act prohibits medical testing of an employee except in circumscribed circumstances. Testing of an employee to determine that employee's HIV status is prohibited unless such testing is determined to be justifiable by the Labour Court.[3] The Act further states that it is *not* unfair discrimination to distinguish, exclude or prefer any person on the basis of an inherent requirement of a job. It is difficult, however, to identify any such situations related to HIV, though there may be such situations identified in future. Thus, employers who believe that knowledge of an employee's HIV status is justified must approach the Labour Court for authorisation before embarking on such testing. In the main, employees with HIV should be treated in the same way as all other employees. This implies that employees with HIV-related illnesses and AIDS should be treated in the same way as employees with other life-threatening illnesses.

Although the Act does provide a prohibition on HIV testing within the employment relationship, an amendment will possibly be introduced during 2000 to define situations where testing is permissible; such as within a patient/health-care worker relationship. A Code entitled *Code of Good Practice on Key Aspects of HIV/AIDS and*

employment, which is to be appended to the EEA, will be promulgated by the end of 2000. This Code's primary objective is to
provide implementation guidelines for employers and employees so
as to ensure that employees with HIV or AIDS are not unfairly dis-
criminated against. It has a secondary objective of providing
guidelines on the management of HIV/AIDS in the workplace.

The testing prohibition

There are presently a range of legal opinions regarding the meaning
of section 7(2) of the Employment Equity Act. These centre around
whether it is an absolute prohibition of HIV testing or not. A *literal*
interpretation of the section is that it forms an absolute prohibition.
This implies that all HIV testing within the workplace is prohibited
unless Labour Court authorisation is obtained. It would not necessarily mean that a company would have to go to court for every
individual HIV test; but broad applications would have to be made,
for example to get authority to run voluntary counselling and HIV
testing (VCT) programmes. Moreover, a single company could apply
on behalf of an entire industry. If authorisation was granted, it would
allow all companies within that industry to run such programmes.

An alternative view is the *nonliteral* one. This is based on a form
of legal interpretation when the meaning of the statute is not clear.
It involves examining the 'intention of Parliament' in drafting the
particular section to determine its meaning. Proponents of this view
argue that only testing which unfairly discriminates is prohibited by
the Act, as Parliament would not have intended the prohibition to
extend beyond this.

Writing in *AIDS Analysis Africa,* Mark Heywood of the AIDS Law
Project[4] explores the interpretation of the Act. He argues that if the
literal interpretation of this prohibition is valid, it will make the
section unconstitutional. This is because an absolute prohibition on
any HIV testing in the context of the workplace would deprive
employees in South Africa of several of their fundamental rights,
particularly their rights to:

■ 'freedom and security of the person',[5] which embraces the common-law right to make personal decisions about health care; and
■ 'access to health-care services',[6] a right which would be violated

should a workplace clinic refuse a request for an HIV test from an employee.

Mark Heywood's interpretation is that the Act is not unconstitutional. It is only interpretations of it that lead to the untenable conclusion that it might be. In fact, the statute states explicitly that it must be interpreted 'in compliance with the Constitution' and 'so as to give effect to its purpose'.[7] That purpose, which is to protect employees with HIV or AIDS from employer-initiated adverse discrimination, clearly licenses employer-funded or employer-provided testing when the employee initiates it.

In the meantime, employers should take reassurance from the words of one of the opinions commissioned by the Department of Labour:

'It is highly unlikely that any legal consequences would flow from an employer offering testing with informed consent and counselling to its employees. It is difficult to imagine what claim an employee who has given informed consent to a test would have (unless that information has been inappropriately circulated or used to discriminate against the employee).'

This opinion may become a touchstone for judging the legality of testing programmes designed to prevent HIV-infected employees from working in conditions which may be conducive to contracting other diseases such as TB, malaria or silicosis. Obviously, the employer may have to offer alternative and less risky career paths for those that test positive. This may not be easy.

Other Acts

In regard to HIV and AIDS, the implications of the other Acts are now examined:

The *Promotion of Equality and Prevention of Unfair Discrimination Act No. 4 of 2000.* This Act does not have a specific section on unfair discrimination in employment, but it does provide in section 5(3) that it will apply if the form of unfair discrimination is excluded from the ambit of the Employment Equity Act.

161

Section 185 of the *Labour Relations Act No. 66 of 1995* (LRA) protects employees against arbitrary dismissal. A dismissal is only fair if it is related to an employee's conduct or capacity or is based on the employer's operational requirements (section 188). All dismissals must be effected with reference to the Code of Good Practice on Dismissals attached to the Act in Schedule 8. This provides that where employees no longer have the capacity to perform their functions, the employer should investigate the following: the extent of their incapacity; alternatives, short of dismissal, such as short-time, extended sick leave without pay; adapted duties; and possible means of accommodating the employee's disability. In this process, employees should be given an opportunity to voice their opinion on the possible alternatives or accommodations. They should be provided with an incapacity hearing before dismissal.

Therefore, a dismissal solely because an employee is HIV positive or has AIDS is likely to be found to be either automatically unfair because it is a dismissal based on discriminatory conduct by the employer or simply unfair if it does not fall into one of the listed categories. However, if an employee who has AIDS-defining illnesses is dismissed for incapacity, it could be fair provided that the steps outlined in the Code of Good Practice on Dismissal have been followed.

The *Occupational Health and Safety Act No. 85 of 1993* (OHSA) requires in section 8(1) that employers, as far as it is reasonably practicable, create a safe working environment. Draft regulations on Hazardous Biological Agents specify what these responsibilities entail. In relation to HIV/AIDS, it is an employer's duty to ensure that steps are taken to assess the risk of occupational HIV infection; that the risk of possible HIV infection is minimised; that appropriate first-aid equipment is readily available to deal with spilt blood and body fluids; that staff training is undertaken on safety steps to be taken following an accident; and that universally accepted infection control procedures are used in any situation where there is possible exposure to blood or blood products. Furthermore, the occupational transmission of HIV/AIDS should be placed on the agenda of companies' Health and Safety Committees to ensure that appropriate control measures are followed.

162

Section 2(1) of the *Mines Health and Safety Act No. 29 of 1996* requires mine owners, as far as it is reasonably practicable, to create a safe working environment. Section 5(1) provides that, in terms of this duty, the mine manager must identify health and safety risks, ensure that employees are not exposed to these risks and supply safety equipment and training. These duties are similar to those in the OHSA which covers other industries and workplaces.

In the *Compensation for Occupational Injuries and Diseases Act No. 130 of 1993* (COIDA), section 22(1) provides for compensation for employees who are injured in the course and scope of their employment, provided that such an injury causes disablement or death. Where an employee becomes HIV infected following an occupational exposure to infected blood or blood products, compensation is possible if the occupational accident can be shown to be the direct cause of the person seroconverting (i.e. becoming HIV positive).

The *Basic Conditions of Employment Act No. 75 of 1997* (BCEA) sets out the minimum employment standards for working hours, leave, etc. The Act states in section 22(2) that every employee is entitled to six weeks paid sick leave within every sick leave cycle. Furthermore, provision is made to negotiate an extension of sick leave but at a reduced rate (provided it is not less that 75 per cent of the ordinary rate of pay). This provision is likely to be important for employees with advanced HIV disease or AIDS.

The *Medical Schemes Act No. 131 of 1998* is a piece of legislation which indirectly affects the employment relationship. The Act regulates Medical Schemes, not employers, but there are implications for employment relationships due to the fact that many employment contracts include some medical cover.

In section 24(2)(e) the Act provides that a medical scheme may not unfairly discriminate, directly or indirectly, against any person on the basis of his or her 'state of health'. Furthermore, in accordance with section 67(1)(g), the Minister of Health is given power to draft regulations stipulating the minimum level of benefits that all schemes

163

must offer to their members. The Act came into operation on 1 September 1999, and medical aid schemes will have a 12-month period to alter their rules to bring them in line with the Act.

Regulations on the *notification of AIDS disease and death* were published for public comment by the Department of Health in 1999. To date the Department has not indicated whether it intends going ahead with these proposals. If promulgated, these regulations would place certain duties on health-care workers including the anonymous reporting of cases of AIDS disease and death and of disclosure to immediate family members, caregivers and those preparing the body for burial.

The Department of Health recently published a draft *HIV testing and informed consent policy* for public comment. The policy sets out the circumstances under which testing may take place and the process which must be followed (which includes informed consent and pre- and post-test counselling). This policy will also apply to HIV testing undertaken within the workplace.

Turning finally to *common-law protection*, every person has rights in terms of the Constitution and common law; these include the right to privacy and bodily integrity. This means that medical treatment (including HIV testing) may only be carried out with the informed consent of the person concerned. The right to privacy also means that individuals are entitled to keep certain personal information to themselves and there is no legal duty on employees to disclose their HIV status to their employer. Moreover, medical practitioners are under a legal and ethical duty to ensure that patient information is not revealed to third parties without consent. This means that information on a person's HIV status may not, in the ordinary course of events, be revealed without consent.

Case study: HIV applicants for employment

The issue of employment in certain jobs and the law on testing have gone to the courts recently. In a High Court case[8] and later a Labour Court case, both heard in Johannesburg, the law grappled with a

164

question which will undoubtedly arise again and again for South African businesses: how to deal with an applicant for employment who is HIV positive. In both cases South African Airways was the employer, but in each case the individual was different.

In 1996 the first individual submitted an application for employment as a flight attendant to SAA. On the strength of his curriculum vitae and various interviews, as well as psychometric tests, he was found to be suitable for the job. The medical examination required by SAA found him to be 'medically suitable'. However, the applicant did not disclose that he was HIV positive, but a routine blood test showed that he was 'an HIV carrier'. SAA then performed a volte-face, and declined to employ him as a flight attendant, offering him alternative employment as a ground staff member instead.

A case was then brought by the applicant under the Constitution. It was heard before Judge Hussein in the Witwatersrand Local Division. The applicant contended that it was an unfair labour practice to refuse to employ him solely on the basis of his HIV-positive status; and that this violated his constitutional rights to dignity, equality, fair labour practices and privacy. However, to prove that the process was 'unfair', he had to show that SAA's actions were arbitrary and irrational.

SAA argued that its policy requires that all flight attendants must be fit for worldwide duty. Flight personnel are therefore obliged to do service on routes to countries which are yellow-fever endemic. They are thus required to be immunised with a live yellow-fever vaccine, which SAA at the time claimed was potentially dangerous for those with HIV infection. Furthermore, in accordance with directives from the Civil Aviation Authority and the Department of Health, SAA is obliged to take all necessary steps to ensure that the health and safety of its passengers are not compromised. Of importance in this regard is that all cabin staff are required to act as safety officers in emergency situations. SAA is therefore obliged not to employ persons with disabilities (such as blindness or epilepsy) who could compromise the safety of passengers in an emergency situation.

Considered as a whole, the court found that SAA's policy was justified and substantiated. The policy is not selectively applied against those persons who are HIV positive. Instead, the policy is directed at detecting all kinds of disabilities which make employment as a flight attendant unsuitable. According to the judge, the 'unsuitability' of a candidate was to be balanced against the policy's considerations of 'medical, safety and operational grounds'. It followed from the above that the court found it justifiable for SAA to conduct medical examinations on aspirant flight attendants, and that the airline's refusal to employ the applicant as a cabin attendant was not an unfair labour practice.

The High Court case raised some difficult questions. Firstly, how does one view an applicant for employment who does not volunteer information about his or her HIV status? What provisions should be in place to protect voluntary disclosure? Secondly, should an AIDS policy not be more specific in its application, making distinctions between those persons who are at different stages of the disease? If the AIDS problem is to be tackled effectively in the workplace, broad policies might have to make way for more specific and principled dealings with the individual concerned. Thirdly, should a business policy be amended so as to be more accommodating of HIV-positive persons? Many of the steps which employers will have to take to accommodate disabled persons (possibly including people with HIV or AIDS) will be detailed in a Disability Code which will be appended to the EEA later in 2000. Could SAA have employed the applicant on routes where yellow-fever innoculations were not required? For example, could he not have been employed internally within South Africa without the need for a vaccination or the threat of exposure to serious diseases? And what is the actual health and safety risk in the event that an attendant is infected with HIV? Finally, how should managerial prerogatives to decide on business policies be balanced with the law?

A very different result emanated from the case brought by the second individual who sought a job with SAA in 1997 and had the same experience in the interview. This case was heard in the Labour Court in May 2000 under the Labour Relations Act. SAA decided to settle out of court. Not only did the company admit unconditionally that the exclusion of the applicant for the post of cabin attendant on the grounds of his HIV status was unjustified; it also paid out

R100 000 compensation and covered all legal costs. Implicit in SAA's admission was the fact that the airline should have obtained its client's informed consent in conducting the HIV test; it should have given the client pre- and post-test counselling in conducting the HIV test; and it should have taken further steps to investigate the extent of the client's immuno-competence.[9] The final point is important because a yellow-fever inoculation may not be harmful to HIV-positive people if their CD4 count is high enough. Moreover, triple-drug therapy may allow them to work normally for many years. SAA also promised to update its policies on HIV and recruitment.

It should be noted that both these incidents occurred before the Employment Equity Act was promulgated. If a case was brought now regarding testing, it would be under the EEA and the court would have to look only at whether or not the testing is *justifiable*. It seems unlikely that general screening for HIV, such as is practised by SAA, will be permissible without Labour Court authorisation. However, notwithstanding the outcome of the second case, authorisation may be given within certain strictly defined parameters.

Conclusion

The case study is not the last word on the issue of HIV-positive job applicants. It is important that those who are involved with the study and research of HIV/AIDS appreciate how difficult it is for the law to deal with the problems associated with the epidemic. This case illustrates some of those difficulties and highlights how far business and the law still have to go towards working out a vision of substantive equality for those with HIV/AIDS.

Existing and new labour legislation provides the legal framework within which workplaces should operate in respect of HIV/AIDS. Organisations should be reviewing their workplace policies, employment practices, protocols and employment conditions to check for compliance with the legislation. In general, if HIV/AIDS is going to be dealt with effectively, employers will need to be more sensitive to the possible ramifications of their business policies and practices. What might have seemed a standard business policy or practice in the pre-AIDS years might now indirectly have the effect of excluding those with AIDS from pursuing their chosen careers.

167

Appendix 3 Useful contacts

AIDS Consortium:
Tel: (011) 403 0265
Fax: (011) 403 2106
Email: *aidscons@global.co.za*
  resource@global.co.za

AIDS Education & Training CC:
Tel: (011) 726 1495
Fax: (011) 726 8673

AIDS Foundation of South Africa:
Tel: (031) 202 9520
Fax: (031) 202 9522
Email: *admin@aids.org.za*

AIDS Law Project:
Tel: (011) 403 6918
Fax: (011) 403 2341
Email: *125ma3he@solon.law.wits.ac.za*

Centre for the Study of AIDS:
Tel: (012) 420 4391
Fax: (012) 420 4395
Email: *nbrummer@ccnet.up.ac.za*

CINDI – Children in Distress – Preparing
for life after AIDS:
Tel: (0333) 45 2970
Fax: (0333) 45 1583
Email: *yspain@pmburg.co.za*
Website: *www.togan.co.za/cindi*

Health Economics & HIV/AIDS
Research Division:
Tel: (031) 260 2592
Fax: (031) 260 2587
Email: *freeman@nu.ac.za*
Website: *www.und.ac.za/und/heard*

Health Systems Trust:
Tel: (031) 307 2954
Fax: (031) 304 0775
Email: *hst@healthlink.org.za*

Hospice Association of South Africa:
Tel: (021) 531 2094
Fax: (021) 531 7917
Email: *hasa@iafrica.com*

Medical Research Council:
Tel: (012) 339 8500
Fax: (012) 339 8582

Medical Research Council – National
AIDS Research Programme:
Tel: (031) 204 3600
Fax: (031) 204 3601

Metropolitan AIDS Research:
Tel: (021) 940 5177
Fax: (021) 940 5678
Email: *skramer@metropolitan.co.za*
Website: *www.metropolitan.co.za*

National AIDS Convention of South
Africa (NACOSA):
Tel: (021) 423 3275
Fax: (021) 423 3274
Email: *nataidc@iafrica.com*

National Association of People with
AIDS (NAPWA):
National office tel/fax: (012) 420 4410

Susan Hyde & Associates:
Tel/fax: (011) 640 7311

Endnotes

1 Understanding HIV and AIDS

1. For an excellent history of the early years of the epidemic, including the search for the virus, see Randy Shilts, *And the Band Played On*, Penguin, London, 1987.
2. The science around the AIDS virus is clearly explained in Christopher Wills, *Plagues, Their Origin, History and Future*, Flamingo, London, 1997.
3. From *www.sirius.com*.
4. Virginia van der Vliet, *New Light on the Origin of AIDS*, published in *PulseTrack*, an electronic newsletter. She quotes a report from B. Korber, 'Timing the Origin of the HIV-1 Pandemic', unpublished paper from the 7th Annual Conference on Retroviruses and Opportunistic Infections, held in San Francisco on 30 January-2 February 2000.
5. Source: The National Institute of Allergy and Infectious Diseases. *www.niaid.hih.gov*.
6. Source: The National Institute of Allergy and Infectious Diseases. *www.niaid.hih.gov*.
7. World Bank, *Confronting AIDS*, Oxford University Press, New York, 1997, p. 59.
8. Taken from the AIDS Brief, *Sports and Physical Activity Sector*, by Prof. M.P. Schwellnus, Sports Science Institute of South Africa, University of Cape Town Medical School, email: *mschwell@sports.uct.ac*. The AIDS briefs have been commissioned by the Health Economics and HIV/AIDS Research Division of the University of Natal under a USAID project. This and the other briefs can be found on the HEARD website, *http://www.und.ac.za/und/heard/*.
9. D. Torre, C. Sampietro, G. Ferraro et al., 'Transmission of HIV-1 Infection Via Sports Injury', *Lancet* Vol. 335 (1990).
10. World Health Organisation (WHO), World Federation of Sports Medicine (FIMS), 'Consensus Statement on AIDS and Sports', *Br J Sports Med* Vol. 23, No. 2, 1989.
11. National Department of Sport and Recreation (South Africa), *Play It Safe: Position Statement on HIV and AIDS*, SISA and SASMA. *'Play It safe'* can be obtained by e-mailing a request, with address and number of copies, to *ezera@sport1.pwv.gov.za*.
12. UNAIDS/Pan American Health Organization/WHO (1998), *Cuba: Epidemiological Fact Sheet on HIV/AIDS and Sexually Transmitted Diseases*, UNAIDS, *www.unaids.org*.
13. Based on: P. Cohen and K. Mitchell, *Long-Term Primary Care Management of HIV Disease*, 1998.

169

14. Prices quoted by LifeSense and Aid for AIDS, 16 May 2000.
15. Most of the data on TB is taken from The Health Systems Trust, *South African Health Review, 1999*, Durban, 1999.

2 The basic epidemiology and data sources

1. J. Katzenellenbogen, G. Joubert and S. Karim, *Epidemiology: A Manual for South Africa*, Cape Town, Oxford University Press, South Africa, 1997.
2. These data are taken from *Epidemiological Comments*, Vol. 22, No. 10, October 1995, Department of Health, Republic of South Africa. This was the last year that AIDS case information was produced.
3. Swaziland National AIDS/STDs Programme, *Sixth HIV Sentinel Surveillance Report, 1998*, Ministry of Health and Social Welfare, Mbabane, Swaziland, September 1998, p. 8.
4. There are two reasonably easy and usable models. The first is a locally developed one from the Actuarial Association of South Africa, *www.assa.co.za*. The second one was developed in the USA by The Futures Group International and is available from *www.tfgi.com/software/spec.htm*.
5. Swaziland National AIDS/STDs Programme, *Sixth HIV Sentinel Surveillance Report, 1998*, Ministry of Health and Social Welfare, Mbabane, Swaziland, September 1998, p. 23.
6. For an excellent discussion on data sources and their value, see UNAIDS Case Study, 'Reaching Regional Consensus on Improved Behavioural and Sero-surveillance for HIV: Report from a Regional Conference in East Africa', UNAIDS *Best Practice Collection*, June 1998:
http://www.unaids.org/publications/documents/epidemiology/determinants/una98e9.pdf.

3 The global epidemic

1. Much of the material for this chapter is drawn from the UNAIDS/WHO, *AIDS Epidemic Update: December 1999*. This document is available from the UNAIDS website: *www.unaids.org.*
2. UNAIDS/WHO, *AIDS Epidemic Update: December 1999*, Geneva, 1999, p. 10.
3. L. Khodakevich, 'Development of HIV Epidemics in Belarus, Moldova and Ukraine and Response to the Epidemics', summary of a presentation at the 8th International Conference on the Reduction of Drug-related Harm, Paris, 23-27 March 1997.
4. The World Bank, Figure 3.11a from Rojanapithayakorn and Hanenburg, 1996, *Confronting AIDS*, Oxford University Press, New York, 1999.
5. The World Bank, *Intensifying Action Against HIV/AIDS in Africa: Responding to a Development Crisis*, Washington D.C., 1999, p. 5.
6. These shocking figures are taken from a 'Memo' issued on 2 June 1999 to World

Bank staff and supporters announcing the new AIDS in Africa initiative: 'A Wildfire is Raging Across Africa'.
7. The World Bank (1999), Statistical Appendix, Table 4: *Confronting AIDS*, Oxford University Press, New York, 1999.
8. Source: The World Bank, *Confronting AIDS: Public Priorities in a Global Epidemic*, Oxford University Press, New York, 1997, p. 87.
9. The World Bank (1999), Statistical Appendix, Table 4: *Confronting AIDS*, Oxford University Press, New York, 1999.

4 The epidemic in South Africa

1. The Department of National Health and Population Development (DNHPD), update, December 1990.
2. The Department of National Health and Population Development (DNHPD), update, December 1990.
3. A. Thom, 'AIDS Looms Large at Province's Hospitals', *Independent Newspapers Online*, 1998, *www.iol.co.za*.
4. J. Vial, 'Survey Finds 2,7m Infected People', *Independent Newspapers Online*, 1998, *www.iol.co.za*.
5. A. Thom, 'AIDS Looms Large at Province's Hospitals', *Independent Newspapers Online*, 1998, *www.iol.co.za*.
6. J. Soal, *Independent Newspapers Online*, 1998, *www.iol.co.za*.
7. D. Beresford, 'The Weak Will Simply Perish', *Mail and Guardian*, 17 February 2000.
8. B. Jordan, 'Johannesburg Reels as AIDS Reaps a Soaring Toll', *Sunday Times*, 28 May 2000.
9. These were areas set aside for the black population of South Africa under the apartheid system. Each 'tribe' was allocated a homeland. Four were 'independent' and six were 'self-governing'.
10. Department of National Health and Population Development, *Epidemiological Comments*, Vol. 19, No. 5, May 1992, Pretoria.
11. S.S. Abdool Karim and Q. Abdool Karim, 'Changes in HIV Seroprevalence in a Rural Black Community in KwaZulu', *SA Med J*, Vol. 82, 1992, p. 484.
12. T. Muhr, using Doyle model of Metropolitan Life, 2000.
13. Compiled by authors from UNAIDS epidemiological comments sheets.
14. UNAIDS and UNICEF have models on the calculation and estimation of the number of orphans on their websites. See *www.unaids.org/hivaidsinfo/software/index.html*.
15. Anthony Kinghorn and Malcolm Steinberg, *HIV/AIDS in South Africa: The Impacts and the Priorities*, Department of Health, 1998.
16. The Futures Group family of models is available from: *http://www.tfgi.com/software/spec.htm*.

5 The severity of South Africa's epidemic

1. Durex Global Sex Survey, 1998, *www.durex.com*.
2. There is also evidence to support this point. In "Children Living with HIV/AIDS in South Africa – A Rapid Appraisal" (see endnote 5 of Chapter 9 for more details), the following excerpt is taken from page 29: "Research with pregnant and non-pregnant teenagers in Khayelitsha, to assess risk factors for teenage pregnancy, found that all the girls (mean age 16,4 years) had had sexual intercourse and at least one boyfiend."
3. From *South African Health Review, 1995*, as quoted in *Epidemiological Comments*, Vol. 1, No. 2, June 1999.
4. UNAIDS/WHO, *Epidemiological Fact Sheet on HIV/AIDS and Sexually Transmitted Diseases, June 1998, www.unaids.org*.
5. Tony Barnett and Alan Whiteside, 'HIV/AIDS and Development: Case Studies and a Conceptual Framework', *The European Journal of Development Research*, Vol. 11, No. 2, December 1999, pp. 200-234.
6. The Gini index measures inequality of income. A Gini index of zero would indicate perfect equality, every person having the same income; and an index figure of 100 would indicate perfect inequality, one person having all the income and the rest having nothing. South Africa's index figure in 1993 was 58,4 compared with Switzerland's 36,1 and the USA's 40,1.
7. South African Government, General Circular No. 25 of 1967.
8. Although these figures may give an impression of spurious accuracy, incredibly detailed records were kept by the Department of Co-operation and Development. For additional information see A.W. Whiteside, 'Some Aspects of Labour Relationships between the Republic of South Africa and Neighbouring States, Part II: Economic Implications', HSRC Investigation into Manpower Issues: *Manpower Studies No. 5*, Pretoria, 1986.
9. The Employment Bureau of Africa Limited, *Report and Financial Statements for Year ended 31 December, 1984, 1989, 1994, 1998*.
10. B. Roberts, 'Apartheid Forces Spread AIDS', *Mail and Guardian Online*, 12 November 1999, *http://www.mg.co.za/mg/za/archive/99nov/12novam-news.html#AIDS*.
11. ISS Monograph Series No. 41, September 1999, *Violence Against Women in Metropolitan South Africa*.
12. Based on *www.rapecrisis.co.za/statistics*.
13. P. Blaikie, T. Cannon, I. Davis and B. Wisner, *At Risk: Natural Hazards, People's Vulnerability, and Disasters*, Routledge, London, 1994, p. 55.

6 Projections and demographic impact

1. These data are taken from Alan Whiteside, 'The Current and Future Impact of HIV/AIDS in South Africa', draft paper prepared for the United Nations Development Programme and submitted in late 1998. The projections were prepared by Thomas Muhr of Metropolitan Life.

2. Based on a projection made with the Doyle model by Metropolitan Life, 1998.

3. K. Michael, C. Desmond and A. Whiteside, *The Impact of HIV/AIDS on Planning Issues in KwaZulu-Natal: A Revisit of the 1995 Report*, draft report prepared for the Town, and Regional Planning Commission of KwaZulu-Natal by the Health Economics and HIV/AIDS Research Division of the University of Natal, 2000.

4. Based on a projection made with the Doyle model by Metropolitan Life, 1998.

5. Based on a projection made with the Doyle model by Metropolitan Life, 1998.

6. Based on a projection made with the Doyle model by Metropolitan Life, 1998.

7. For the most recent and complete review of the thinking on this topic see Michel Carael, and Bernhard Schwartlander (editors), 'Demographic Impact of AIDS', *AIDS*, Vol. 12, Supp. 1.

8. J.A. Adetunji, 'Assessing the Mortality Impact of HIV/AIDS Relative to Other Causes of Adult Deaths in Sub-Saharan Africa', the Socio-Demographic Impact of AIDS in Africa Conference, International Union for the Scientific Study of Population, and the University of Natal, Durban, February 1997. Also J.T. Boerma, J. Ngalula, R. Isingo, M. Urassa, K. Senkoro, R. Gabone and E.N. Mkumbo, 'Levels and Causes of Adult Mortality in Rural Tanzania with Special Reference to HIV/AIDS', the Socio-Demographic Impact of AIDS in Africa Conference, International Union for the Scientific Study of Population, and the University of Natal, Durban, February 1997.

9. Y.J. Bryson, 'Perinatal HIV-1 Transmission: Recent Advances and Therapeutic Interventions', *AIDS*, Vol. 10, Supp. 3, 1996, pp. S33-S42.

10. United States Bureau of the Census, *World Population Profile, 1998*, Population Division International Programme Centre, Washington D.C., 1998.

11. United Nations, Human Development Reports, Oxford University Press, New York, 1996, 1997 and 1998. Note that the life expectancies used for calculating the human development index are for 1993, 1994 and 1995 respectively.

12. S. Gregson, Tom Zhuwau, Roy M. Anderson and Stephen K. Chandiwana, 'HIV and Fertility Change in Rural Zimbabwe', and Lucy M. Carpenter, Jessica S. Nakiyingi, Anthony Ruberantwari, Samuel S. Malamba, Anatoli Kamali and James A.G. Whitworth, 'Estimates of the Impact of HIV Infection on Fertility in a Rural Ugandan Population Cohort', *Health Transition Review*, Vol. 7, Supp. 2, 1997.

13. J. Stover and P.O. Way, 'Impact of Interventions on Reducing the Spread of HIV in Africa: Computer Simulation Applications', *African Journal of Medical Practice*, Vol. 2, pp. 110-120.

14. J.P.M. Ntozi, 'Widowhood, Remarriage and Migration during the HIV/AIDS Epidemic in Uganda', the Socio-Demographic Impact of AIDS in Africa Conference, International Union for the Scientific Study of Population, and the University of Natal, Durban, February 1997.

15. Produced by T. Muhr, 1999.

16. Produced by T. Muhr, 1999.

17. Quoted in a brief prepared for the Cabinet of KwaZulu-Natal by Karen Michael of the University of Natal Health Economics and HIV/AIDS Research Division, Durban, 1998.

18. Ministry of Welfare and Population, White Paper on Population Policy, Pretoria, March 1998.

7 The economic, developmental and social impact of AIDS

1. Keith Edelston, *AIDS: Countdown to Doomsday*, Media House Publications, Johannesburg, 1988.
2. Mead Over, 'The Macroeconomic Impact of AIDS in Sub-Saharan Africa', Africa Technical Department, Population, Health and Nutrition Division, Technical Working Paper No. 3, Washington D.C., June 1992.
3. See for example I.T. Cuddington, 'Modelling the Macro-economic Effects of AIDS, with an Application to Tanzania', *World Bank Economic Review* 7, 1992, pp. 403-417; L. Forgy and A. Mwanza, *The Economic Impact of AIDS in Zambia*, Ministry of Health, Lusaka, 1994; and G. Kambou, S. Devarajan and M. Over, 'The Economic Impact of AIDS in an African Country: Simulations with a Computable General Equilibrium Model of Cameroon', *Journal of African Economics* 1, 1992, pp. 109-130.
4. Sapa, 'HIV/AIDS "to stunt" Botswana's economy', *Business Day*, 16 May 2000.
5. World Bank, World Development Reports, various years, Oxford University Press, New York.
6. The Centre for Health Policy, 'AIDS in South Africa: Demographic and Economic Implications', Department of Community Health, University of the Witwatersrand, Johannesburg, Paper No. 23, September 1991.
7. Ibid, p. 71.
8. Department of Finance, *Budget Review 2000*, Pretoria, 2000, p. 40.
9. Ibid, p. 29.
10. ING Barings, South African Research, 'Economic Impact of AIDS in South Africa: A Dark Cloud on the Horizon', Johannesburg, April 2000.
11. J. Katzenellenbogen, 'AIDS to Slash South Africa's Growth' and 'World Leaders to Get AIDS Wake-up Call', *Business Day*, 11 and 12 April 2000.
12. Szu Fuei Chong, 'A Critical Review of Household Survey Methodology: Assessing the Cost Effectiveness of Household Responses to the Economic Impact of HIV/AIDS', Masters dissertation, School of Development Studies, UEA, Norwich, 1999.
13. The main sources for this very large-scale study are: M. Ainsworth and M. Over, 'Measuring the Impact of Fatal Adult Illness in Sub-Saharan Africa: An Annotated Household Questionnaire', Living Standard Measurement Working Paper No. 90, World Bank, Washington, 1992; M. Ainsworth, L. Fransen and M. Over, 'Confronting AIDS: Evidence from the Developing World', the European Commission, Brussels and the World Bank, Washington D.C., 1998; G. Koda and M. Over, 'The Cost of Survivor Assistance Programs in Northwestern Tanzania', Int-Conf-AIDS, 6-11 June 1993, Vol. 9, No. 2, p. 926 (abstract no. PO-D29-4250); M. Over, P. Mujinja, M. Ainsworth, G. Koda, I. Semali, G.

174

Lwihula, and I. Gupta, 'Economic Impact of Adult Death from AIDS: Overview of preliminary results from a Random Sample of Households in Tanzania', Int-Conf-AIDS, 6-11 June 1993, Vol. 9, No. 2, p. 918 (abstract no. PO-D28-4200), together with the data which have been reported in *Confronting AIDS: Public Priorities in a Global Epidemic*, World Bank, Oxford University Press, Oxford, New York, 1997.

14. World Bank, *Confronting AIDS*, 1997, pp. 208-9. Op. cit.
15. P. Kwaramba, 'The Socio-economic Impact of HIV/AIDS on Communal Agricultural Systems in Zimbabwe', Working Paper No. 19, Economic Advisory Project, Friedrich Ebert Stiftung, Harare, 1998.
16. W. Janjareon, 'The Impact of AIDS on Household Composition and Consumption in Thailand', N. Bechu, 'The Impact of AIDS on the Economy of Families in Côte d'Ivoire: Changes in Consumption Among AIDS-affected Households', R. Menon, et al., 'The Economic Impact of Adult Mortality on Households in Rakai District Uganda', all in Ainsworth, Fransen and Over, op. cit.
17. This glaringly obvious point was first made by Prof. Tony Barnett at a meeting attended by one of the authors in Belgium in 1996.
18. Communication from R. Harbour, University of Natal, 2000.
19. This is discussed in a number of recent publications, see for example World Health Orga-nisation Department of Health in 'Sustainable Development, Health in Poverty Reduction', Collected Papers, mimeo (undated) and Department for International Development, International Development Target Strategy Paper, Consultation Document, 'Better Health for Poor People', DFID, London, November 1999.
20. H.R. Gabriel, 'Rugalema, Adult Mortality as Entitlement Failure: AIDS and the Crisis of Rural Livelihoods in a Tanzanian Village', PhD thesis, Institute of Social Studies, The Hague, Netherlands, September 1999.
21. J. May (editor), 'Poverty and Inequality in South Africa', report prepared for the office of the Executive Deputy President and the Interministerial Committee for Poverty and Inequality, Paxis Publishing, 1998.
22. Stefan de Vlyder, Issue Paper on Socio-economic Causes and Consequences of HIV/AIDS, SIDA Health Division Document, Stockholm, 1999, p. 3.
23. For a full discussion of the development impact of AIDS see Tony Barnett and Alan Whiteside, 'HIV/AIDS in Africa: Implications for "Development" and Policy', paper presented at the Standing Committee on University Studies of Africa, Fourth SCUSA Interuniversity Colloquium, 5-8 September 1999.
24. United Nations Development Programme 1999, *Human Development Report 1999*, Oxford University Press, New York, p. 1.
25. Robert D. Putnam with Robert Leonardi and Rafaella Y. Nanetti, *Making Democracy Work: Civic Traditions in Modern Italy*, Princeton University Press, Princeton, 1993.
26. Stats SA, October Household Survey, 1998. *www.statssa.gov.za*.
27. UNAIDS, *Children Orphaned by AIDS*, *www.unaids.org/unaids/events/wad/1997/orphan.html*, 12 May 1999.

28. Martin Schönteich, 'AIDS and Age: SA's Crime Time Bomb', *AIDS Analysis Africa*, Vol. 10, No. 2, August/September 1999.

29. M.M. MacKay, 'AIDS will Spur on Crime Say Experts', *Saturday Argus*, Cape Town, 9 January 1999.

30. L. Sergal, J. Pelo and P. Rampa, 'Asicamtheni Magents. Let's Talk Magents', *Youth Attitudes towards Crime and Conflict*, University of Natal, 15.24, Autumn 1999.

8 AIDS and the private sector

1. It is particularly telling that in the search for information for a UNAIDS-supported three-country study of best practices, there was a real problem in identifying a range of best practices in South Africa. See Dr R. Loewenson et al., *Best Practices: Company Actions on HIV/AIDS in Southern Africa*, Organisation of African Trade Union Unity, Harare, February 1999.

2. John Stover and Laurie Bollinger, 'The Economic Impact of AIDS', The Futures Group International, unpublished paper, Glastonbury, USA, 1999.

3. Matthew Roberts and Bill Rau, *African Workplace Profiles: Private Sector AIDS Policy*, AIDSCAP, Arlington, VA, USA.

4. The published brochure is a summary of the report prepared by Drs Malcolm Steinberg and Gill Schierhout of Abt Associates South Africa Inc. for Anglo American plc. For further information, telephone (011) 638 3176.

5. C. Jones, 'The Micro-economic Implications of HIV/AIDS', MA thesis, School of Development Studies, University of East Anglia, Norwich, 1996.

6. Dr Chester N. Morris and Dr Edward J. Cheevers, 'The Direct Costs of HIV/AIDS in a South African Sugar Mill', *AIDS Analysis Africa*, Vol. 10, No. 5, February/March 2000.

7. The April 1998 edition of the *AIDS Bulletin*, a publication produced by the Corporate Communications Division of the Medical Research Council, took as its theme 'HIV/AIDS in the Workplace'. The publication includes articles on company response, AIDS and the law, employment equity, and so on, but only *one* article makes reference to the impact.

8. Karen Michael, 'HIV/AIDS and the Retail Sector', *AIDS Analysis Africa*, Vol. 9, No. 6, April/May 1999.

9. This was presented at a meeting for clients organised by AMB-DLJ Securities in Cape Town in February 2000.

10. To this end, the JD Group has announced, subject to various conditions, the R2 billion share-funded acquisition of Ellerines, another large furniture and appliance retailer in South Africa. See A. Crotty, "Ellerine's Buy Will Make JD Group JSE's Biggest Retailer", *Business Report*, 10 May 2000.

11. This work is drawn from a study being carried out by the Harvard Institute for International Development with a number of South African partners. The models presented here are from a chapter in a book, *HIV/AIDS in the Com-*

monwealth, published by Kensington Publications in conjunction with the Commonwealth Secretariat, London. The chapter is by Jonathan Simon, Sydney Rosen, Alan Whiteside and Jeffrey R. Vincent and is entitled 'The Response of African Businesses to HIV/AIDS'.

12. The Lesedi Project, 'A Success Story: STD Interventions Prevent HIV', mimeo 28 June 1999.

9 AIDS and nation building

1. J. Rademeyer, Zubeida Jaffer and SAPA-AFP, "AIDS Rivals Devise Ways to Settle Dispute," *The Star*, 8 May 2000.
2. The production of these toolkits has been co-ordinated by the Health Economics and HIV/AIDS Research Division (HEARD) of the University of Natal. The local government toolkit was developed by Rose Smart, former head of the AIDS Directorate in Pretoria, with support from the KwaZulu-Natal provincial government and USAID. The government toolkits were developed by Abt. Associates and HEARD with support from USAID. The documents can be found at the HEARD website, *www.und.ac.za/und/heard*.
3. A. Shevel, 'Talks Held on Pfizer's Offer of Free AIDS Drug', *The Star*, 3 May 2000.
4. S. Barber, "AIDS Drug Prices Slashed', *Business Day*, 12 May 2000.
5. A rapid appraisal of children infected with and affected by HIV/AIDS was commissioned in October 1999 by the Interim National HIV/AIDS Care and Support Task Team (NACTT), funded by Save the Children (UK). The rapid appraisal seeks to provide information for the national strategy and the various national, provincial and local processes emanating from it. 'Children Living with HIV/AIDS in South Africa: A Rapid Appraisal', written by Rose Smart is available from Save the Children Fund's South African office in Pretoria, telephone (012) 341 1889.
6. The National Intelligence Council, *The Global Infectious Disease Threat and its Implications for the United States*, USA, January 2000.

10 The challenge of AIDS for South Africa

1. Published in *The Citizen*, 20 April 2000.
2. David R. Patient and Neil M. Orr, 'What Teenagers and Young Adults Have to Say about Condoms and Using Condoms', *AIDS Analysis Africa*, Vol. 10, No. 6, March/April 2000.
3. Metropolitan Life and Department of Health.
4. Estimate by Gary Taylor of Medscheme, March 2000.
5. Figures quoted by Dr André van Bassen, LifeSense Disease Management (Pty) Ltd, 16 May 2000.
6. 'Children Living with HIV/AIDS in South Africa: A Rapid Appraisal', by Rose Smart.

7. Stephen Morgan, 'Response for All AIDS Affected Children, Not AIDS Orphans Alone', *AIDS Analysis Africa*, Vol. 10, No. 6, March/April 2000.

Appendix 1 Treatment options

1. G. Gray, 'Anti-retrovirals and Their Role in Preventing Mother to Child Transmission of HIV-1', *The Implications of Anti-retroviral Treatments*, WHO and UNAIDS, 1998.
2. E. Marseille, J. Kahn, F. Mmiro, L. Guay, P. Musoke, M. Flower and J. Jackson, 'Cost Effectiveness of Single-dose Nevirapine Regimen for Mothers and Babies to Decrease Vertical HIV-1 Transmission in Sub-Saharan Africa', *The Lancet*, Vol. 354, 1999, pp. 803-808.
3. Ibid.
4. A. Kinghorn, 'Projections of the Cost of Antivetrovirals Interventions to Reduce Mother to Child Transmission of HIV in the South African Public Sector', HIV Management Services: Johannesburg, 1998.
5. M. Mascolini, 'Conference on Treatment of the HIV Infection: Sharing the Data, Shopping for Wisdom', *Journal of the International Association of Physicians in AIDS Care*, Vol. 5, No. 11, 1999, pp. 17-26.
6. N. Soderlund, K. Zwi, A. Kinghorn and G. Gray, 'Preventing Vertical Transmission of HIV: A Cost Effectiveness Analysis of Options Available in South Africa. *British Medical Journal*, Vol. 318, 1999, pp. 1650-1656.
7. E. Marseille, J. Kahn, F. Mmiro, L. Guay, P. Musoke, M. Flower and J. Jackson, 'Cost Effectiveness of Single-dose Neviropine Regimen for Mothers and Babies to Decrease Vertical HIV-1 Transmission in Sub-Saharan Africa', *The Lancet*, Vol. 354, 1999, pp. 803-808.

Appendix 2 The legal framework and HIV/AIDS

1. This appendix was largely written by Rose Smart, HIV/AIDS consultant, and Ann Strode, HIV/AIDS and law consultant. It was originally researched and developed for the Placer Dome Western Areas Joint Venture. Parts of it were published in *AIDS Analysis Africa*, Vol. 10, No. 3.
2. The Act also provides that should a dispute arise between different statutes, then the provisions the EEA will prevail.
3. Testing to establish an employee's HIV status is expressly prohibited. Medical testing is defined in the Act as any test, question, inquiry or other means designed to ascertain, or which has the effect of enabling an employer to ascertain, whether an employee has any medical condition.
4. M.J. Heywood, 'HIV Testing in the Workplace: Clarifying the Meaning of South Africa's Employment Equity Act', *AIDS Analysis Africa*, Vol. 10, No. 6.
5. The Constitution of the Republic of South Africa Act 108 of 1996, s 12(2).

6. Ibid, s 27(1). Although this right may be limited and is dependent upon available resources, it is unimaginable that a court would accept that a severe limitation of this right could be justified on the grounds that the health service was found on the premises of an employer.
7. Ibid, s 3 (a) and (b).
8. This is taken largely from Max du Plessis, 'Applicants for Employment who are HIV-Positive: A Recent Case', AIDS Analysis Africa, Vol. 11, No. 1.
9. A. Shebel, 'SAA Admits to Poor HIV Policy and Offers R100 000 to Job Applicant', Business Report, 11 May 2000.